1987

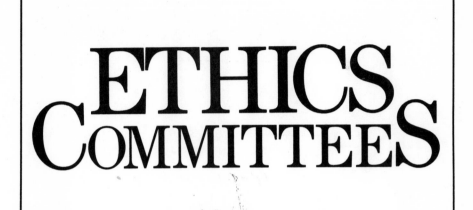

ETHICS COMMITTEES

A PRACTICAL APPROACH

ETHICS COMMITTEES

A PRACTICAL APPROACH

Robert P. Craig, EdD
Carl L. Middleton, DMin
Laurence J. O'Connell, PhD, STD

Copyright © 1986
by
The Catholic Health Association of the United States
4455 Woodson Road
St. Louis, MO 63134-0889

Printed in the United States of America.

Library of Congress Cataloging-in-Publication Data

Craig, Robert Paul.
  Ethics committees.

  Bibliography: p.
  Includes index.
  1. Medical ethics. 2. Ethics committees.
3. Catholic health facilities. I. Middleton, Carl L.
II. O'Connell, Laurence. III. Title. [DNLM: 1. Ethics,
Medical. 2. Pastoral Care. 3. Professional Staff
Committees. 4. Religion and Medicine. W 50 C886e]
R725.3.C73   1986   174'.2   85-28020
ISBN 0-87125-110-8

Contents

v

Introduction

As the health care environment grows more and more complex, the need for collaboration on a variety of issues is undeniable. Rapid technological advances, limited resources, and a socioeconomic climate characterized by cost containment concerns are demanding that providers reflect more consciously on the nature of health care and how it is to be delivered. Within the broad range of concerns presently demanding attention, ethical issues are among the most prominent. This is to be expected, since the present socioeconomic, political situation is forcing choices on the general public as well as on providers in health care. And ethics is all about choices. Ethics aims at developing a reasoning process or method for deciding what ought to be done in the face of ambiguous choices, that is, in the face of alternative ways of acting that are inconsistent and logically incompatible in some sense. Will placing a patient on a respirator extend that person's life or will it unnecessarily delay death? Choices: Here we have the meat of ethics.

In response to the growing need to make hard choices, many health care institutions have recognized a need to develop a formal mechanism to come to terms with the ethically charged, rapidly shifting dynamics of health care delivery today. The so-called institutional ethics committee (IEC) is emerging as the preferred means of dealing with ethical dilemmas. The IEC seems to offer at least an interim answer to the demand for ethical sensitivity in the provision of health care.

In *Ethics Committees: A Practical Approach*, we attempt to provide a clear description of the nature and function of the IEC. Admittedly this is one approach among potentially many, but it is, in our opinion, broadly applicable and generally representative of what is happening in the field. Although certain passages do address specifically Roman Catholic concerns, this book is designed for anyone interested in learning more about IECs.

This book aims at offering a concise, well-informed discussion of the practical aspects of planning and implementing an ethics committee in acute care as well as continuing care institutions. Moving from a general consideration of the who, what, and why of the IEC, the discussion then focuses on the dynamics of ethical decision making. We also offer a model for the initiation and continuing education of the IEC. Some chapters are followed by practical exercises that allow readers to apply and clarify its content immediately.

━━━━━chapter one

Why Ethics Committees?
What Can They Do?

Background

Recent interest in ethics committees is rooted in three significant events in the area of health care, namely, the Karen Quinlan case (1976), the recommendations of the President's Commission for the Study of Ethical Problems in Medicine and Biomedical and Behavioral Research (1983), and finally the circumstances surrounding the promulgation of the so-called Infant Doe regulations (1984-1985). Institutional ethics committees (IECs) had been used sporadically for several years, but the combined impact of the foregoing events prompted many individuals and organizations to undertake systematic studies of the benefits, functions, and problems of IECs.

The Quinlan and "Baby Doe" cases as well as the very existence of a presidential commission are symptomatic of conditions inherent in contemporary culture that tend to focus attention on ethical considerations in health care. Richard McCormick has delineated eight cultural variables or background conditions that are presently promoting interest in ethics committees:

1. *The complexity of problems.* "With the growing sophistication of medical technology and the expansion of treatment options, the ethical and medical dimensions of many decisions have become indistinct and complex. Since both health care personnel and health care institutions presumably wish to engage in 'ethically acceptable' practices, they begin to look for help in gray areas."

2. *The range of options.* In trying to determine the 'best interest' of patients, there may well be a range of acceptable behaviors. "It has become increasingly clear that such a determination exceeds the perspective of an individual and that a group [e.g., an ethics committee] might be expected to approximate more nearly [even if not always achieve] the 'reasonable person standard'."

3. *Protection.* "Decisions are much less likely to be [legally] contested if they have the backing of an ethics committee, for the decision will be seen to surpass individual [possibly idiosyncratic and 'interested'] perspectives and very likely to conform to public standards of the acceptable."

4. *Nature of judgments in clinical decisions.* Today it is recognized that competencies other than medical expertise affect clinical decisions. "We have become newly aware of this in recent years, and that awareness is the backdrop for the emergence of interdisciplinary ethics committees."

1

5. *The emergence of patient autonomy.* Conflicts between patients and physicians or health care institutions often require the type of mediation and arbitration an ethics committee can offer.

6. *The emergence of economic considerations.* As economic resources begin to dwindle, decisions will have to be made concerning who gets how much health care.

7. *Religious convictions of some groups.* Religiously sponsored health facilities need a forum for discussing their ethical and religious standards in reference to medical practice.

8. *Individual decisions as affected by the plurality of publics.* "Decision making is no longer simply a one-on-one affair. Increasingly, health care personnel must be responsible to a variety of publics, Medicare and Medicaid agencies, group practice sensitivities, religious policies, state or federal legislation.... Some of the values for which these publics stand compete with each other. Resolution of such conflicts may not be achieved through medical or scientific judgments; rather, such resolutions call for policy decisions that range far beyond medical expertise."[1]

Given the complexity of the health care environment, ethics committees can serve several significant purposes.

Functions

The description of cultural conditions that underlie the widespread emergence of ethics committees does more than point to a general need; it also suggests specific functions for IECs. The four general functions for IECs are education, development of policies and guidelines, consultation and case review, and, under certain circumstances, theological reflection.

Education

IECs should begin with self-education by familiarizing themselves, both theoretically and practically, with the relevant issues. Committee members will find a growing body of pertinent literature as well as an increasing availability of conferences, seminars, correspondence courses, etc., designed specifically to meet their needs. The Catholic Health Association (CHA) maintains a list of current publications and activities.

Experts testifying before the President's Commission enumerated several dimensions of an IEC's educational function:

First, in ethics committees with a diverse membership of physicians, nurses, other professionals, and lay people, discussions allow the various members to share perspectives and views, which can lead to better decisions regarding the treatment .... Of particular importance here is the way ethics committees can expose the actual decision makers in a hospital setting to various ethical and social considerations.

Second, over a period of years ethics committees may provide a setting for people within medical institutions to become knowledgeable and comfortable about relating ethical principles to specific decisions.

Third, presenting a number of issues through actual cases that receive institutional attention is likely to underscore the seriousness of the issues involved, the possibility of better and worse resolutions, and the obligations of all to address the issues responsibly.

Finally, ethics committees may serve as a focus for community discussion and education, which is likely to stimulate thought beyond issues of incompetence to a consideration of more general bioethical issues.[2]

Thus, IECs are seen as having several educational roles in medical decision making. Taking the educational function a step further, Sr. Margaret Farley has suggested that the IEC educational role should extend beyond bioethical and medicolegal questions to social justice issues in health care:

"Social justice" refers to questions not only of respect for individual patients (for their safety, their autonomy, their general well-being), but of fairness to patients in relation to other patients and to society. It has to do with the allocation of scarce resources, the fair distribution of benefits and burdens, and the rights of members of a human community to participate in decisions that affect their lives. It concerns primarily the structures and processes that allow the just distribution of power, the protection of human rights, and security for the weak and vulnerable.[3]

Sr. Farley contends that IECs should educate themselves and others on these critical issues as they affect health care delivery in a particular institution. A number of practical considerations would seem to argue against extending the educational function of the IEC to social justice issues, but it is certainly worthy of consideration as a committee shapes its agenda.

Development of Policies and Guidelines

The President's Commission called for clear-cut policies regarding decisions affecting patients who lack adequate decision-making capacity. As R. E. Cranford and A. E. Doudera have noted, "This is a role for which ethics committees seem highly suited and one which many committees have performed."[4]

Cranford and Doudera, however, envision an even broader role for the IEC in the era of policy development. The IEC, for instance, might also "propose, review, and recommend to the hospital, administrative policies and guidelines on such problems as the determination of death, orders not to resuscitate, foregoing life-sustaining treatment, supportive care, and treatment of handicapped newborns. Moreover, in conjunction with its educational role, the committee could review guidelines and policies in light of the newest information."[5]

3

Thus, "the multidisciplinary ethics committee is especially well suited to the task of developing and revising general policies or guidelines" as well as "...overseeing the implementation of newly developed institutional guidelines."[6]

Consultation and Case Review

The IEC may serve in a consultative role during an ethically complicated case. The committee or its members might review the case in an effort to help patients, family, the medical staff, et al., surface, understand, and respond to a broad range of ethical and social concerns. "The committee would serve as a resource with specialized training, understanding, and experience within the institution—be it a hospital or nursing home—for staff and families."[7]

The President's Commission has suggested a more judgmental role for the IEC in the area of case review, recommending that the committee actually decide whether or not treatment decisions in specific cases lie within the range of permissible alternatives. "This type of involvement is controversial and has, in fact, been rejected in many ethics committee charters."[8] We would agree with those who suggest that IECs "not be final decision makers but that they strive to emphasize the role of the attending physicians and surrogates as the primary decision makers . . . ."[9] This, of course, would not preclude the possibility of an IEC initiating judicial review under certain extreme circumstances.

Finally, the whole notion of the IEC undertaking retrospective review of cases should be carefully considered, since the "spectre of after-the-fact faultfinding may be counterproductive to the committee, reducing medical staff cooperation, as well as leading to a 'watchdog' approach implying a duty of care on the part of the committee."[10]

This is not to say that retrospective review is an entirely inappropriate exercise of the review function. When retrospective review is undertaken, however, the review's purpose must be clearly specified. Any form of "witch hunting" is inappropriate.

Theological Reflection

Theological reflection is directed toward understanding one's faith tradition. As St. Anselm noted, theology is faith seeking understanding. Within a Catholic health care facility's context, an IEC can contribute to the understanding of the Roman Catholic faith tradition as it encounters the cultural variables already mentioned. Within the IEC the religious and ethical convictions of Roman Catholicism both challenge and are challenged by contemporary developments. The role that an IEC can play in developing the Roman Catholic moral tradition is treated in some detail later. Here it is sufficient to note that a religiously affiliated health care facility can expect its IEC to function as a vehicle for its religious self-understanding, either directly or indirectly.

Problems

Although an IEC is generally recognized as a valid and oftentimes very effective institutional response to problems with decision making, it also gives rise to a variety of problems. The problems should be recognized and squarely faced.

Among the most prevalent problems associated with IECs is physician resistance. Physicians have been accustomed to going it alone. In commenting upon an IEC's possible role, a well-known professor at Johns Hopkins Medical School remarked: "In 30 years of practice, I never had a case that I could not handle on my own."[11]

Some physicians consider the IEC a threat to their professional autonomy and authority as well as an affront to their personal integrity. Physicians are concerned that IECs will inappropriately insinuate themselves into the privacy of the patient-physician relationship. Increasingly, however, physician resistance is subsiding as wary practitioners gradually learn that the IEC is much more a help than a hindrance.

Confidentiality is another problem. What right does a committee, perhaps drawn from nonprofessional personnel within the hospital and even the general public, have to review a patient's highly personal medical records? "Hospital staff cannot presume that patients have consented to a display of their cases before such a group, especially if the disclosure involves details of their private lives."[12] Thus an IEC must make a concerted effort to guarantee confidentiality. For instance, if confidential patient information is used in committee discussions, any minutes or case notes should be recorded in such a way as to guarantee patient anonymity.

Institutional self-interest gives rise to other concerns. Understandably, IECs might be tempted to look after the interests of their colleagues and the institution they serve. "Obviously, an attitude of in-house protectionism can affect the quality of ethical deliberation and the ultimate credibility of an ethics committee."[13] If, however, an IEC understands and accepts its mission, this should not become a significant issue. Other questions will inevitably arise in discussing an IEC's pros and cons:

- How and when does an IEC engage in "whistle blowing?" Is it ever appropriate?
- How does an IEC weigh the respective demands of law and ethics? Although something may be legal, it may not be ethical.
- How does an IEC do justice to the pluralism that characterizes our society? How can it adapt to cultural and religious differences?
- How does the IEC overcome the lack of ethical expertise or medical knowledge among its members?
- How will the ethics of the IEC itself be developed?

The experience of several IECs has already demonstrated that none of the foregoing problems is insurmountable. Yet, as Fr. McCormick wisely counsels, "the institutions that establish ethics committees would do well to weigh them in advance, to circumvent unnecessary opposition and possibly obstacular tactics."[14]

Footnotes

1. Richard A. McCormick, "Ethics Committees: Promise or Peril?" *Law, Medicine, and Healthcare*, September 1984, pp. 150-152.
2. President's Commission for the Study of Ethical Problems in Medicine and Biomedical and Behavioral Research, *Deciding to Forego Life-Sustaining Treatment*, U.S. Government Printing Office, Washington, DC, 1983, p. 163.
3. Margaret Farley, "Institutional Ethics Committees as Social Justice Advocates," *Health Progress* October, 1984, p. 32.
4. R.E. Cranford and A.E. Doudera, *Institutional Ethics Committees*, Health Administration Press, Ann Arbor, MI, 1984, p. 16.
5. Ibid., p. 16.
6. Ibid., p. 16.
7. Ibid., p. 16.
8. Ibid., pp. 16-17.
9. Ibid., p. 17.
10. *Legal Issues and Guidance for Hospital Biomedical Ethics Committees*, American Hospital Association, January 1985, p. 7.
11. Cranford, p. 91.
12. McCormick, p. 153.
13. Ibid., p. 154.
14. Ibid., p. 154.

━━━━━━━━━ chapter two

The Who and The What of Ethics Committees: Membership and Structure

Membership

The composition of institutional ethics committees (IECs) has been the subject of some debate. The discussion primarily focuses on exclusivity vs. inclusivity. For example, if an IEC serves solely as a prognosis committee, as in the Quinlan case, it might seem reasonable to limit membership on the committee to physicians. If, however, it serves more general purposes, as we are suggesting, the membership should reflect these broader purposes. If, for instance, an institution has decided that the IEC is to fulfill the broad range of functions described in Chapter One, the IEC's membership will necessarily be quite diverse.

This should not be taken as an endorsement of diversity for diversity's sake. As Alexander Capron has said:

> Instead, institutional officials ought to decide whether they intend to bring in a cross-sample of the community in order to replicate the sort of choice that a jury would make if this were a case that had gone to court. Alternatively, are they seeking diversity to obtain additional insights into technical questions (including the technical issues of ethics)?—in which case one would want a professor of philosophy or a theologian or whatever is necessary. In any case, my message is: decide why it is that you are looking for individuals other than physicians to be decision makers. Do not answer the 'who' question with diversity for its own sake, but because of the specific functions you want diversity to serve. [1]

Depending on the institution's needs and size, a typical committee might include administration, trustees, physicians from various specialties, nurses, social workers, patient representatives, members of the pastoral care team, lawyers, and theologians/ethicists, as well as lay persons from the general public. Nominations for the IEC often but not always come from department heads, whereas the administrator makes the formal appointment in most cases. Other methods of nominating and appointing can and probably should be explored.

Special problems are associated with three potential IEC members: the lawyer, the person from the pastoral care department, and the representative of the general public.

The role of the lawyer must be clearly understood:

> A hospital may decide that the attorney who represents the hospital should act as a member of the committee in order to provide legal perspective to committee deliberations when necessary; however, care should be taken to avoid any possible conflict of interest inherent in this arrangement. Another view is that it may be difficult for an attorney to both advise the committee and act as a member. This view would then prompt a structure with an attorney member of the committee chosen from the community, and the hospital's attorney as counsel. It may be unwise for the committee to have its own attorney since it may appear that the committee is not representative of the hospital.[2]

Thus, if a lawyer serves on or relates to an IEC, his or her role must be carefully defined and appropriately structured.

Because of the close link between religion and ethics, the pastoral care department's representative is often singled out as the most likely candidate to chair the IEC. This sometimes leads to complications, since it often seems to convey the idea that the IEC focuses primarily on spiritual or religious issues. As we shall later see, religious factors can significantly influence an IEC, but the IEC incorporates far more than religious considerations in its deliberations and activities. Thus, given the potential for misunderstanding, it is probably best not to select someone from pastoral care as the IEC's chairperson.

Finally, the role of lay persons from outside the health care facility may present some problems. On the one hand, some critics contend that inviting members of the general public to serve on an IEC may increase the chances that the patients' right to confidentiality will be violated. On the other hand, it has been argued that the presence of community representatives keeps institutions and IECs honest by guarding against the sort of in-house protectionism mentioned earlier. Moreover, lay persons serve as liaisons between the technical, clinical world and the world of ordinary persons with no special expertise.

Each institution must weigh the relative advantages and disadvantages of including the general public, depending on its own situation. For example, a small, rural hospital may find it more difficult to include lay persons on an IEC than a large, urban medical center, since it is less likely that individual patients would be known to IEC members in a large metropolitan area. Whenever possible, however, lay persons should be included.

In arguing in favor of lay persons' membership, Leonard Glantz makes a valid point:

> When we consider the composition of institutional ethics committees, we generally think about physicians, clergypeople, nurses, lawyers, and social workers. As a result, such committees will tend to be white, middle-class, and profoundly over-educated. They will be people who value and are concerned about intellectual life .... It seems to me that if the committees are going to make decisions for handicapped people, we should try to involve people who have some

of those handicaps. In this manner, we can avoid making assumptions about the meaning and impact of conditions which we have not experienced. Having blind, deaf, wheelchair-bound, and mentally retarded members will make these committees more representative of the people whom their decisions will affect.[3]

Glantz would support the point of view that, although lay persons may not be permanent members of a given committee, they should at least be involved on an ad hoc basis, depending on the issue under discussion. The President's Commission for the Study of Ethical Problems, in its argument supporting a diverse membership for an IEC, also promotes this point of view: " . . . many different perspectives should be available so that the advice can be communicated in a way that speaks to the varied needs and orientations of patients and practitioners."[4]

Initial Formation

Once an institution is committed to forming an IEC, it is essential that the administrator organize an educational program concerning the committee. All hospital personnel should be well informed about the committee's background, goals, and functions before it is formally constituted. The IEC is directed toward improving the quality of the decision-making process throughout the facility, so its workings should be given high visibility and the administrator's support should be seen as unequivocal.

Following the introductory educational program and the committee's appointment, IEC members should focus on self education, familiarizing themselves with their task and the resources available to them, both internally and beyond the institution. Members should be encouraged to share their understanding of the committee and what they as individuals can offer. Also, at this point the clinicians must begin to translate their technical language into ordinary terms, while nonclinical members must try to familiarize themselves with clinical attitudes and language. This may be difficult, but failure to do so will ultimately undermine the ability of committee members to communicate with one another.

The committee should begin by discussing procedural matters (e.g., meeting dates and times, attendance of alternates or substitutes, quorum requirements, use of subcommittees) and some of the ethical issues they will probably face (e.g., informed consent, resource allocation, withdrawal of life-sustaining treatment, advance directives, do-not-resuscitate orders). The committee should concentrate on its educational and policy formulation functions *before* initiating its consultative function, if it chooses to offer consultation services at all.

Initial meetings should be directed toward allowing committee members to get acquainted with one another. Gradually, as the trust level in the group grows, the committee will be prepared to move into discussing substantive issues. The familiarization process should not be forced or rushed. Social gatherings after meetings often are helpful.

Given the need for a certain level of trust and open exchange, it is best to limit the IEC to 8 to 12 members at any given time in an average size institution. Terms should be staggered to establish a rotating membership. The committee should meet once a month and begin promptly at the appointed time, since tardiness can seriously erode morale, especially in a health care setting where demands on time are notoriously intense.

Structure

The IEC's specific structure will dictate the scope of its responsibilities and the extent of its accountability. Thus the way in which an institution chooses to structure its IEC will determine the limits of the committee's authority and accountability.

Three structural models for the IEC have been suggested: optional/optional, mandatory/optional, and mandatory/mandatory.[5] Each model assigns a range of responsibility and accountability to the IEC, moving from responsibility for simple consultative services with relatively limited accountability to responsibility for complex decision making with significant accountability, both within and outside the institution. There are arguments in favor of each model.

By the optional/optional form, we mean that "the physician [or other concerned party] has the option of consulting with the committee on ethical matters, as well as the option of choosing whether to follow its advice."[6] Thus the IEC functions in a strictly consultative capacity and has no decision-making authority of its own. It does not assume responsibility for the actions of the health care team, patients, or families. Since the optional/optional IEC serves simply as an advisory body for health care team members, its accountability, especially legal liability, would be quite limited. In fact, many states have statutes that would probably provide immunity from legal liability for an optional/optional IEC.

Although the optional/optional structure does provide a forum for addressing the moral issues and conflicts that increasingly come to the fore in clinical practice, there are drawbacks to this approach. When referral to the IEC is merely optional, for example, it may well be ignored. "Achieving the goals and functions of an institutional ethics committee requires that cases be brought to it. Thus, leaving this decision optional...will result in IECs being greatly underutilized.... Data about existing ethics committees confirm this fear."[7] Thus, if decision making in all areas of ethical concern is to be enhanced, the IEC may have to be structured along more authoritarian lines in some situations.

It has been suggested that: "Whenever there is likelihood that a clinical decision will implicate important nonmedical interests the physician and family or patient should not have the sole right to decide."[8] For example, sterilization of retarded persons, bone marrow or other transplants from minors, and the treatment of imperiled newborns are considered by some as cases for mandatory review. For example, "while many physicians or hospitals may refuse to sterilize a retarded person without a court order, a less costly alternative to judicial review would be review by an IEC to ascertain whether the sterilization can in fact be justified as being in the retarded person's interests."[9]

Thus, "the scope of mandatory review depends upon a prior value judgment of the relative importance of the interests at stake and the likelihood that competing interests may skew the results of clinical judgments."[10]

If an institution decides that its IEC will at times function as a forum for mandatory review, it must also decide whether a mandatory/optional or a mandatory/mandatory process is desirable. Will the physician, for instance, be required to bring certain cases (a child with Down's syndrome and an uncomplicated intestinal obstruction) to the IEC for review, yet not be bound to follow the committee's recommendation (mandatory/optional)? Or, will review *and* compliance with the IEC's recommendations be required (mandatory/mandatory)? This question is still being debated. Some contend that the crux of the problem lies in defining "those cases in which review should be mandatory, and where ultimate decisional authority is given to the ethics committee."[11]

Although in some highly specialized areas (e.g., neonatal intensive care), some form of mandatory review may be warranted, we believe that the IEC itself should never be given *"ultimate decisional authority."* In cases where substantive disagreement between the IEC and other principal parties persists, the committee should follow established procedures to report its conclusions to the hospital authority responsible for reporting such cases to the appropriate civil agency or court. In short, the mandatory/optional model may serve in certain specific contexts, but the mandatory/mandatory model is not well suited to an IEC as we envision it.

Thus, in a manner consistent with what we said regarding the committee's consultative function, we would strongly recommend against characterizing the IEC as a decision-making body. Among other problems, "the potential legal implications of such a role include conflict with patient autonomy, appearance of the corporate practice of medicine and the strong possibility of more judicial involvement." Moreover, "there are also questions of greater procedural burdens regarding, for example, access and appeals to the committee records."[12]

An IEC's position within the institutional hierarchy is very important. Health care facilities, as with all large organizations, have a recognizable power structure that should be taken into account when assigning an IEC its place on the institutional flow chart. Ideally, the IEC should be associated with either the medical staff committee, the administration/hospital committee, or whatever are the most prominent committees. Identification with these influential forces will ensure the IEC the kind of support and visibility it needs. Genuine support from the administration and medical staff are essential if the IEC is to fulfill its mission successfully.

Footnotes

1. Alexander Capron, as quoted in R.E. Cranford and A.E. Doudera, *Institutional Ethics Committees*, Health Administration Press, Ann Arbor, MI, 1984.
2. *Legal Issues and Guidance for Hospital Biomedical Ethics Committees*, American Hospital Association, January 1985, p. 13.
3. R.E. Cranford and A.E. Doudera, *Institutional Ethics Committees*, Health Administration Press, Ann Arbor, MI, 1984, p. 134.
4. Ibid., p. 181.
5. John A. Robertson, as quoted in R.E. Cranford and A.E. Doudera, *Institutional Ethics Committees*, Health Administration Press, Ann Arbor, MI, 1984.
6. Ibid., p. 91.
7. Ibid., p. 90.
8. Ibid., p. 92.
9. Ibid., p. 92.
10. Ibid., p. 92.
11. Ibid., p. 93.
12. *Legal Issues and Guidance for Hospital Biomedical Ethics Committees*, American Hospital Association, January 1985, p. 7.

chapter three

Religious Perspectives and Ethical Choices

As an institutional ethics committee (IEC) grapples with ethical dilemmas arising from difficulties in such areas as institutional policy formulation, individual medical practice, and shared social responsibility, many forces will affect the committee's deliberations. This chapter addresses one significant factor which can and often does affect the process of ethical decision making, namely, religious perspective.

In fact, the impact of religious perspectives on moral judgment gives rise to a crucial issue for an IEC, especially in a religiously affiliated health care institution: How does an IEC respectfully accommodate the moral perspectives of nonbelievers as well as believers of different faith traditions? For instance, is it possible—and if it is possible, is it desirable—for a Catholic long term care facility to invite nonbelievers and representatives from other faith traditions to serve on its IEC? The answer is a resounding, YES! But why? Parenthetically, we should note that our response to this question will be fashioned against the background of the Roman Catholic theological tradition.

Christians affirm a general unity of authentic human morality which goes beyond any single religious perspectives. Thus, Christians contend that moral consciousness or conscience is a characteristic quality of *all* women and men. Thus, "in fidelity to conscience, Christians are joined with the rest of men in the search for truth, and for the genuine solution to the numerous problems which arise in the life of individuals and from social relationships."[1]

Regardless of how one characterizes the specific nature of Christian morality, it must be emphasized that "it does not and cannot add to human ethical self-understanding as such any material content that is, in principle, 'strange' or 'foreign' to [persons] as [they] exist and experience [themselves] in the world."[2] This, of course, is not to deny that Christian faith informs the personal moral consciousness of believers. It is a simple assertion of the radical congeniality of all moral consciousness. Once this has been established it is possible to approach the specific character of Christian morality in a manner which recognizes its inherent continuity with the ethical self-understanding of all persons while still doing justice to its uniqueness.

The Roman Catholic Perspective

Although our work is designed to provide a practical approach to the formation and continuing education of IECs in general, we also have a specific interest in Roman Catholic health care facilities and the problems they face in developing IECs. Thus, it is important at this point that we address moral judgment from a specifically Roman Catholic point of view. While we hope to clarify the dynamics of ethical decision making for Roman Catholics themselves, our comments may also serve to acquaint those who are not Roman Catholic with the type of religious perspective they will encounter if they join an IEC at a Catholic institution.

Catholics, like all Christians, believe that whoever follows Christ, the perfect human being, becomes more fully human. Christ revealed the in-depth meaning of the human way of being. That was his Gospel, his Good News. Thus, Christians believe that in looking at Christ we are looking at humanity par excellence. Perfection is standing before us, concretized in the person of Christ. Christians are called to imitate this objective standard, to mirror this perfect human person in their moral judgments and actions. If a Christian's judgments and actions are inconsistent with the witness of Christ, they are less fully human.

Thus, Catholics believe that they have been given a specific insight, an enlarged perspective on human existence which they feel duty-bound to bring to bear upon ethical questions. This accounts for the distinctive attitudes and intentions which Catholics, most Christians for that matter, bring to discussions of ethical issues. This attitude rests upon the conviction that

> "...because the resources of Scripture, dogma, and Christian life are the fullest available 'objectification' of the common human experience, the articulation of man's image of his moral good that is possible within historical Christian communities remains privileged in its access to enlarged perspectives on man."[3]

Again it must be emphasized that since Christian ethics is the objectification in Jesus Christ of what every person experiences subjectively, "it does not and cannot add to human ethical self-understanding as such any material content that is, in principle, 'strange' or 'foreign' to [persons] as [they] exist and experience [themselves] in the world."[4] Further, it should be noted that, although Jesus Christ was the perfect human being, Christians may not yet have uncovered every feature of this humanity. Non-Christians may well have discerned certain noble features of the human way of being which Christ may have exhibited but which have gone unnoticed by his professed followers. Thus, although Christians do have privileged access to enlarged perspectives on the human way of being, other persons or religions may also enjoy other forms of authentic insight. In fact the Catholic Church rejects nothing that is true and holy in these. "She regards with sincere reverence those ways of conduct and of life, those precepts and teachings which, though differing in many aspects from the ones she holds and sets forth, nonetheless often reflect a ray of that Truth which enlightens all persons."[5]

Ethical Style

Members of an IEC in a Catholic facility should be familiar with the sources which the Roman Catholic tradition draws upon in evaluating and responding to the ethical implications of human activity. How do Roman Catholics generate the enlarged perspective on human existence which ideally guides their personal and institutional moral development? What criteria do they draw upon to ensure the propriety of their moral judgments? How do Catholics address the more or less typically problematic situations of human life which demand judgments, decisions, and oftentimes, hard choices?

The ethical style of Roman Catholicism is characterized by reliance upon normative sources of moral insight. These sources may be subsumed under three general categories: (1) Sacred Scripture and Tradition, (2) Personal Experience, both individual and communal, and (3) Culture. Catholics believe God operates in and through all three sources. The dialectic relationship, that is, the give and take among these sources accounts for ever deepening insight into the cognitive, affective, and moral dimensions of the human person as revealed in Jesus Christ. The interaction of the three sources generates the enlarged perspective on human experience which, as mentioned earlier, informs the ethical style of Roman Catholics.

Again the practical thrust of this book neither demands nor recommends an in-depth study of the sources of moral insight within the Roman Catholic Tradition. This would involve a lengthy digression which in the present context does not seem warranted. However, a few remarks regarding each source as it may relate to the work of IECs are in order.

Sacred Scripture and Tradition

The Bible, which is comprised of the Hebrew Scriptures (Old Testament) and the Christian Scriptures (New Testament) is the pre-eminent source of moral insight for Catholics. "Scripture remains not only an excellent but an incomparable source and norm," since it is through the Scriptures that we encounter Christ, the exemplar, in a most intimate manner.[6] Thus, in dealing with difficult situations of human life or formulating policies for a Catholic health care facility, an IEC must take into account the normative character of Sacred Scripture.

Sacred Scripture, however, is not the sole source of moral insight. "Tradition is another one of its sources and norms and there is real development..."[7] Catholics are not biblical fundamentalists, that is, they do not always take the written word of the Bible literally. For example, *Genesis*, the opening book of the Bible, states that the world was created in seven days. Catholics would contend that the biblical account of creation in *Genesis* is not necessarily to be taken literally. Catholics believe that the biblical account of creation is meant to convey a religious truth, not necessarily historical fact: we are creatures who owe our existence to a caring Creator. Whether or not the world was created in precisely seven days is not the point. In brief, Sacred Scripture is primarily directed towards expressing truth rather than providing historical facts in the empirical sense. Truth can be expressed in myth, allegory, parable, etc., as well as through historical accounts.

According to Catholics, Tradition is the medium or vehicle through which the truth expressed in the Bible is developed or seen more deeply. The Catholic tradition is open to development which, although guided by Scripture, moves beyond a literal reading of biblical texts. Scripture always remains something greater and more comprehensive than the written word; it is "a principle constantly giving rise to new development which it pervades and governs."[8] Similar to the deepening ethical insight which accompanies personal moral development, the tradition as a whole progressively develops and deepens its insight into its biblical foundations. Tradition, as the on-going source of deepening insight, must be considered in confronting moral dilemmas.

Recognizing the relationship between Scripture and Tradition as sources of moral insight within Roman Catholicism is potentially very important to members of an IEC. It is likely that many IECs in Catholic facilities will draw upon the insights of Christians who are not Roman Catholic. Some of these Christians, coming from fundamentalist traditions, will exhibit a personal moral consciousness which is shaped by a literal understanding of the Bible. Some Jews and other non-Christians may also be inclined to interpret the Hebrew and Christian Scriptures in a literal sense. The resulting difference in moral perspective can be significant. Such differences are certainly acceptable, yet it may facilitate discussion if IEC members come to terms with these differences early in the formation of the committee.

Personal Experience

Today Roman Catholicism is characterized by an openness to ordinary lived experience—both individual and communal—as a central and trusted source of moral insight. Unfortunately, this sensitivity to personal experience was lost for some time; but this is neither the time nor the place to describe the long history of Roman Catholicism's recovery of lived experience as a significant factor in the development of moral consciousness.[9] The upshot of this recovery is, however, relevant to our discussion of IECs, especially in Roman Catholic facilities.

Recognition of personal experience as a legitimate locus of God's unfolding revelation, highlights the fact that individual Christians, as well as the Christian communities they comprise, have to enter into the tradition; they have to make it their own. Tradition is not something merely existing "out there" or "back there" with which persons have to deal. Tradition also resides within persons. Thus, "they have to rethink it for [themselves] by a kind of personal application equal to that of [their] predecessors who shaped it in the course of time."[10] Consequently, contemporary moral consciousness cannot go back; it can only go forward consciously extending the on-going impetus of the Judeo-Christian tradition.

An IEC in a Catholic health facility serves the Tradition as a whole by facilitating thoughtful consideration of contemporary moral dilemmas and seeking to resolve them in a manner which exhibits consistency with the tradition while doing justice to the contemporary context. Genuine respect for the personal experience of IEC members, whether Catholic or not, is therefore essential since the IEC serves as one, albeit very tiny, context where the Judeo-Christian tradition engages the actual experience of twentieth century women and men. Respect for personal experience as a source of moral insight under-girds the view that moral tradition is not laid on; it is lived out!

Cultural Context

The ethical style of Roman Catholicism also incorporates a keen awareness of culture. "It is a fact bearing on the very person of man that he can come to an authentic and full humanity only through culture, that is, through the cultivation of natural goods and values. Wherever human life is involved, therefore, nature and culture are quite intimately related."[11] Catholicism is quite comfortable in acknowledging the positive values of today's general culture.[12] For instance, although the dangers of technology are noted, the positive value of technology is continuously supported. Catholicism is also committed to preserving the particular features of the different individual cultures which make up the human family, including their unique moral values.[13]

An IEC, then, should be aware of the broad cultural context within which it is working. The highly developed state of medical technology in the United States, for instance, will have a bearing on the discussion of ethical dilemmas. Although the positive value of technology is readily acknowledged, the ethical style of Catholicism demands that its uses be carefully scrutinized. Simply because something is technically possible does not necessarily mean it is ethically acceptable.

Beyond the broad cultural context lies a full range of specific cultural concerns which an IEC should recognize. Although the substantive ethical dilemma under consideration may be fairly common to all parts of the country and in all segments of the population, the resolution of that dilemma should be handled with sensitivity to the cultural background of the individuals or communities involved. For example, an orthodox Jewish individual or a predominantly Native American community will have unique perspectives on certain medical issues which should be an integral component of the IEC's discussion. Ethical dilemmas in health care always take shape within a cultural context and sometimes *because* of the particularities of specific cultural settings. Roman Catholicism's respect for distinctive cultural values in the formation of moral perspectives should thus be an integral component in the work of an IEC in a Catholic facility, especially in cross-cultural settings like the southwestern United States, certain regions in Canada, or in urban areas where there are large ethnic or racial subcultures.

Summary

Religious consciousness and the perspectives it generates will often be prominent, especially in religiously affiliated health care facilities. The religious perspectives of IEC members and their institution, as well as the religious point of view of those who relate to the committee, will often come into play. The ethical style of Roman Catholicism, for example, will inevitably affect ethical discourse in Catholic institutions. The reliance of Catholicism upon Sacred Scripture and Tradition, personal experience, and culture as valuable sources of moral insight will significantly impact the work of an IEC. In the following chapter we shall expand upon the influence of the specifically Roman Catholic perspective.

Footnotes

1. W.M. Abbott, *Documents of the Second Vatican Council*, Corpus Books, New York, 1966, p. 214.
2. James F. Bresnahan, SJ, "Rahner's Christian Ethics," *America*, 123: 1970, pp. 351-354.
3. Ibid.
4. Ibid.
5. Gregory Baum, *The Teachings of the Second Vatican Council*, The Newman Press, Westminster, MD., 1966, pp. 268-269. 268-69.
6. Karl Rahner and Herbert Vorgrimler, *Theological Dictionary*, Herder & Herder, New York, 1965, p. 55.
7. Ibid., p. 55.
8. Ibid., p. 65.
9. Laurence O'Connell, "Karl Rahner: Human Experience and Theology," *Theology Digest*, (314): 337-393, 1984.
10. H. Walgrave, *Unfolding Revelation*, Westminster, Philadelphia, 1972, p. 390.
11. Abbott, p. 259.
12. Ibid., pp. 263-264.
13. Ibid., pp. 260.

Workshop Exercise

Rather than move through a formal exercise, it is best to provide an opportunity for each member of the IEC to share his or her religious convictions and briefly explain how their religious perspective influences their personal decision making. Nonbelievers should also be given an opportunity to explain how they make ethical choices and which factors they consider in achieving ethical insight.

chapter four
The History and Role of the Ethical and Religious Directives

The development of the Roman Catholic moral perspective through reflection on Sacred Scripture and tradition, personal experience, and culture is guided by what is called the magisterium or the Church's authoritative teaching function. Thus Catholic tradition develops according to neither the accepted notions of public opinion nor the whims of individual preference at a given point in history. It is authoritatively guided in a manner that ensures its consistency with Sacred Scripture and post-biblical Church tradition. Richard McBrien provides a brief description of the Church's teaching authority:

> In the *widest sense* of the term, *teaching authority belongs to the whole Church.* The Second Vatican Council taught that the whole People of God participates through Baptism in the threefold mission of Christ as Prophet, Priest, and King . . . . In the *more restricted sense, magisterium applies to particular groups of teachers whose authority is grounded in their office* (as in the case of the pope and bishops) *or in their scholarly competence* (as in the case of theologians) . . . . In the *strictest sense* of all, however, the term *magisterium* has been *applied exclusively to the teaching authority of the pope and the bishops.*[1]

Although it is generally recognized that the entire People of God share in the Church's teaching function, it must be stressed that the duty to teach authoritatively is "conspicuous among the principal duties of bishops."[2] It is an essential feature of their pastoral office. They are specifically called to teach on such matters as "the human person with his freedom and bodily life, the family and its unity and stability, the procreation and education of children, civil society with its laws and professions, labor and leisure, the arts and technical inventions, poverty and affluence."[3]

The bishops play a central role in the development of Catholicism's moral tradition by virtue of their authoritative teaching function. Not surprisingly, then, the bishops feel duty-bound to comment on moral issues affecting health care delivery. This is particularly true in a health care environment that is presently struggling with those aspects of moral life pertaining to many of the concerns that the bishops are specifically called to address: "the human person with his freedom and bodily life" (e.g., patients' rights, surrogate decision making, organ transplants), "family and its unity and stability" (e.g., chemical dependency, care of the elderly, child and spouse abuse), "the procreation of children" (e.g., abortion, artificial insemination, in vitro fertilization, genetic counseling, genetic experimentation) "civil society with its laws" (e.g., the inequities of Medicare/Medicaid, legal battles over "wrongful life," do-not-resuscitate orders, criteria for establishing clinical death), and technological inventions (e.g., the rapid growth of health-related technologies).

Ethical and Religious Directives for Catholic Health Facilities

The American bishops have exercised their responsibility for communicating the ethical and religious values of Catholic tradition within the context of health care by publishing a national code that sets forth some basic norms delineating the moral responsibility of Catholic-sponsored health facilities. This code is known as the *Ethical and Religious Directives for Catholic Health Facilities* and is subject to each bishop's approval for use in his own diocese.

The *Directives* strive to give expression to the Church's self-understanding of its mission and to read the "signs of the times" by providing direction for Catholic health care institutions in their efforts to carry on Christ's healing mission.[4] According to Joseph Cardinal Bernardin, the *Directives* "flow from our deepest convictions about life, its sacredness, and our obligation to heal and care for it in the best possible way."[5] So the *Directives* represent the bishops' effort to bring the moral and religious values of Roman Catholic tradition to bear on contemporary health care.

Development

The present edition of the *Directives* published in 1971 and slightly revised in 1975, represents several decades of reflection on ethical and religious issues in health care in the United States and Canada. In 1918 Rev. Michael P. Bourke, director of hospitals for the Detroit diocese, drafted the first ethics code, which consisted of a list of ethical standards. Although the Catholic Hospital Association (CHA) of the United States and Canada had some reservations about its completeness, it decided to accept and publish the code. It appeared in the first volume of *Hospital Progress* in 1920. The CHA viewed this initial attempt more as a means of stimulating further reflection on the ethical aspects of health care than a definitive code, since Rev. Bourke's work was very narrowly focused: "To one reading this original code, it becomes quite evident that the main consideration centered on the ethical aspects of surgical operations that involved abortion."[6]

The need for a more comprehensive ethical code was the subject of seemingly endless discussion. After 1920 several dioceses began to draft codes of their own to keep pace with theology and medical technology. The dioceses of Hartford, Toledo, Grand Rapids, and Los Angeles were among the first to develop ethical codes. The *Toledo Code* was recommended to other dioceses and hospitals by the National Catholic Welfare Conference, an agency of the U.S. bishops.

Although the CHA had difficulty in developing a definitive code, in 1935 it did succeed in publishing a document that outlined the basic moral principles on which a Catholic hospital was founded. "The document was a definite step forward in that it went well beyond the exclusion of certain surgical procedures. It emphasized the primary objective of hospitals: the adequate care of the patient."[7] Finally, in 1949, under the sponsorship of CHA, the *Ethical and Religious Directives for Catholic Hospitals* were published. In 1954 a condensed form of the *Ethical and Religious Directives* was published as the *Code of Medical Ethics for Catholic Hospitals*. This soon became the official code in many dioceses in the United States and Canada. A revised version of the *Directives* was issued in 1955. No major changes were considered for several years.

By 1965, however, the press of socioeconomic and political conditions, rapid advances in medical technology, and the enlightened theological perspectives of the Second Vatican Council demanded that the *Directives* be reexamined. Many hospital administrators called on the CHA to initiate a formal review process.

The steady stream of requests for a restudy of the *Directives* prompted the CHA Council on Research, Education and Development to ask the CHA board of trustees to seek the guidance of the American bishops. The U.S. Catholic Conference responded by establishing a commission on Church Health Services to study the problems arising from the *Directives*. The commission first studied the issue of whether the board of trustees of a voluntary, not-for-profit hospital had the right to restrict or prohibit certain medical procedures or services that are accepted legal and medical practice. The Commission upheld the private hospital's right to restrict such procedures on ethical grounds. This position has been upheld by the courts.[8]

After the study's legal phase had been completed, the commission proceeded with the theological study of the *Directives*. A special panel of five theologians and medical resource personnel concluded that the present set of *Directives* posed serious ethical dilemmas for Catholic hospital administrators. They suggested that a revised set be written that would emphasize the concern of Catholic health care facilities for excellence at all levels of quality health care delivery. They said this concern should reflect the Gospel of Christ, the meaning of the healing ministry, suffering and death, and total patient care. A report was submitted to the American bishops on completion of the study's legal and theological phases.

In September 1969, the Board of the U.S. Catholic Conference directed the Committee on Health Affairs to make formal recommendations for consideration by the bishops in the revision of the *Ethical and Religious Directives*. A team of three theologians was asked to draft a revision for the committee's consideration: Richard McCormick, SJ, John R. Connery, SJ, and Paul E. McKeever.

Upon completion, a draft of the proposed revision was submitted to the committee, which in turn referred it to the National Conference of Catholic Bishops' Committee on Doctrine for discussion and approval. In February

1971 the episcopal members of the Committee on Health Affairs received comments and suggestions from their fellow bishops. In order to study these suggestions more fully, an official vote was delayed until the November 1971 meeting. The revised *Directives* were finally approved by the United States Catholic Conference by a vote of 232 to 7, with 2 abstentions. It should be noted that the final revised *Directives* were not based upon the work of the McCormick-Connery-McKeever committee which had been virtually dismissed.

This in part probably accounts for the fact that the new *Directives* met with some sharp criticism from several quarters, most notably a number of highly respected American theologians. Consequently, the Catholic Theological Society of America (CTSA) appointed a study commission in June 1971. The report of the CTSA study group was accepted by the CTSA board of directors on Sept. 1, 1972 and published in the November 1972 issue of *The Linacre Quarterly*. This critical study was "not presented as the final word on codes of ethics for Catholic hospitals, but [was] proposed as a moral theological rationale for understanding the purposes and functions of a set of ethical directives in Catholic hospitals, and as a basis for dialogue, research, and the revision and interpretation of policies."[9]

The CTSA study commission concluded that the *Directives* needed further development since they did not address several relevant topics that, in the authors' opinion, deserved more research and dialogue within the Church. The following are some of the topics that the commission thought required more attention:[10]

1. The Catholic hospital's service to the poor and underprivileged
2. The ethics of power in the Catholic hospital, especially as this relates to the control over medical services by the medical profession, the "consumer," etc., and the determination of fees
3. Quality of health care in Catholic institutions as an ethical issue
4. Racial segregation and discrimination
5. A just family wage, educational and career advancement opportunities, and the other benefits that can rightly be expected from employment in Catholic health facilities
6. Clearer guidelines on the right to die in dignity, the prolongation of human life, the definition of "extraordinary means" for preserving life, the ethics of medical heroics, and the understanding of death as part of life
7. The importance of obtaining informed consent and the efforts required from the professionals involved
8. Transplantation: informed consent, use of children as donors, etc.
9. Human experimentation: safeguards, informed consent, use of children in experimentation, etc.
10. Genetic counseling: its necessity, its limitations, limits on "right to procreate" vs. freedom of choice
11. The extent of the rights of the retarded to be cared for in a manner commensurate with their needs

the CTSA commission urged that steps be taken toward a
the 1971 *Directives*: "Procedures should be established for
tematic revision, which should involve all of the pertinent

e has been no substantial revision of the 1971 *Directives*,
ps are clearly open to such revision. The preamble of the
Directives clearly states that the bishops or their representatives "should regularly receive suggestions and recommendations from the field, and should periodically discuss any possible need for an updated revision of the *Directives*."[12] This is consistent with the bishops' special responsibility for teaching and developing the moral values of the Catholic tradition through reflection on Sacred Scripture and tradition, personal experience, and culture.

Institutional ethics committees (IECs) can do much to assist in the development of the Catholic moral perspective in health care. IEC members can certainly bring personal and cultural experience to bear upon the Church tradition.

Specific Functions

A set of ethical directives or a code of ethics can have several functions, all related to a group's understanding of good decision making and behavior in a particular context. A code of ethics may be:

- *Instructional*—providing moral and ethical information to the uninformed
- *Declaratory*—declaring the group's values, goals, and objectives to its own members and others;
- *Conservative*—upholding certain essential standards of behavior that conserve the group's unity and identity
- *Policy Setting*—providing a definite method of action to guide and determine decisions and to evaluate behavior once the decisions have been taken
- *Arbitrational*—enunciating principles and establishing or allowing for procedures for the resolution of conflicts of consciences
- *Coercive*—creating varying degrees of social pressure or sanction to guarantee adherence to a certain ethical behavior and to provide both internal and external identification

In short, then, "a code is a statement of values, an assertion of goals, and/or an expression of rules whose purposes all focus on good decision making and behavior."[13] The American bishops have sought to fulfill these purposes in varying degrees by issuing a national code. This is entirely consistent with their teaching role and the special responsibility they bear for guaranteeing the perpetuation and development of the moral values of Catholic tradition.

An ethical code's general purposes, as just outlined, help clarify the specific functions of the *Directives* which may be grouped under six headings:

communication, conservation, facilitation, evaluation, arbitration, and protection.

Communication

The primary function of the *Directives* is the perpetuation and development of the moral and religious values of the Roman Catholic tradition in health care. The *Directives* are both instructional and declaratory. They provide moral and ethical information to hospital personnel, patients, families, and the community. Moreover, the *Directives* declare some central values that delineate the goals and objectives of a Catholic health care facility. For example, the holistic orientation of Catholic health care is clearly stated in the preamble: "The total good of the patient, which includes his higher spiritual as well as his bodily welfare, is the primary concern of those entrusted with the management of a Catholic health facility."[14]

Conservation

The *Directives* are also directed toward upholding certain essential standards that conserve a Catholic institution's identity. In reflecting on this point, Cardinal Bernardin noted that unless Catholic institutions "implement the kind of specific values these directives provide, the institutions as corporate persons will become ethically and morally neutral or secular."[15] Present concern for maintaining the specifically Catholic identity of our health care institutions would seem to support the notion that the present *Directives* be further developed, since certain key moral values within Catholic tradition are not explicitly addressed. A fuller exposition of Roman Catholic moral values vis-a-vis the contemporary health care environment in the United States and Canada will highlight the distinctive character of Catholic health care ministry.

Facilitation

The *Directives* facilitate ethical decision making by shaping the context of ethical discourse. "They should not be looked upon as merely a checklist of dos and don'ts."[16] They are guides to the implementation of Catholic value principles in the more or less typically problematic health care situations that demand judgments, decisions, and often hard choices. Again, the rapidly changing dynamics of health care, coupled with the enormous improvement in medical technology in the last 10 years, seems to recommend a reevaluation of the general scope of the *Directives* since their focus is presently very specific.

Evaluation

The *Directives* also serve as a criterion for evaluating professional behavior and the quality of service within the health facility. Thus the *Directives* are one means of guaranteeing adherence to ethical behavior consistent with a Catholic-sponsored institution's mission.

Arbitration

The *Directives* provide a resource for mediating differe
both within the health care facility and in its dealings with th
instance, in dealing with a difficult case that has divided the
IEC may find the *Directives* helpful in reaching a solutic..
parties, while at the same time exhibiting sensitivity to the institution's value
orientation.

Protection

The *Directives* also serve a Catholic health facility in relating to a plural-
istic social situation:

> The empirical fact of pluralism pervades every major dimension of
> our lives—intellectual, cultural, social, ethical and religious—and it
> provides the context for today's healing ministry of the Church. We
> are now being challenged to determine what our response to plural-
> ism should be—how we should articulate the impact our pluralist
> setting in America has on the mission of the Catholic hospital and
> on the way in which ethical norms for these hospitals should be
> explicated.[17]

The *Directives* can help settle cases resulting from conflicts between
Catholic moral values and the moral perspectives of other groups and individuals in society.

For example, Catholic hospitals have not been immune from pressures
to permit abortion on demand, although direct abortion is contrary to Catholic moral teaching. To date, attempts to force them to allow abortions have
been uniformly unsuccessful. It has been demonstrated that no statutory or
common law basis for a court order exists that says a Catholic hospital must
permit abortion.

The *Directives* have been cited in court cases as clear evidence that a
Catholic hospital's refusal to allow abortions is directly attributable to the
ethical and religious convictions of its sponsors. Thus the *Directives* provide
legal protection for Catholic moral and religious values. Consequently it has
been recommended that a Catholic health care facility have "a corporate and
administrative structure that assures adherence to the *Directives*" as a means
of ensuring that the available constitutional and statutory protections are not
inadvertently negated."[18] In short, the *Directives* have proved to be secure
grounds for a legal defense of the Catholic ethical perspective in a court of
law. Although legal protection is certainly not a primary function of the
Directives, it is worth noting.

Institutional Ethics Committees and the *Directives*

The *Ethical and Religious Directives for Catholic Health Facilities*
should be understood as one element in a comprehensive moral and dogmatic

tradition. It represents an attempt to bring specific aspects of that larger tradition to bear on health care delivery in the United States today. (The same can be said for the Canadian Catholic Medico-Moral Guide). The *Directives* as with Catholic tradition as a whole, flow from the interaction of the three sources of moral insight already mentioned in Chapter Two: Sacred Scripture and tradition, personal experience, and culture.

In that the *Directives* share in the larger tradition, they can be expected to exhibit Catholic tradition's developmental character:

> God has completed his self-communication in Christ. But revelation is not only something that proceeds from God. It has to be received in the human mind. The process through which the mind of the Church is penetrated by the Word of God, leading to a progressive understanding of all its implications, can go on as long as history lasts.[19]

Just as the Roman Catholic tradition as a whole is open to progressive understanding of the truth, so also are all expressions of the tradition. Thus the *Directives* must be open to development. This is clearly recognized in the preamble to the *Directives* "...the United States Catholic Conference, with the widest consultation possible, should regularly receive suggestions and recommendations from the field, and should periodically discuss any possible need for an updated revision of these *Directives*."[20]

The emergence of IECs is indeed a blessing. What better forum for the discussion of complicated health care issues as they relate to Catholic tradition? IECs are in a unique position to respond to the bishops' request for suggestions and recommendations from the field. An IEC's multidisciplinary membership provides for depth through the many competencies represented as well as practicality through its intimate involvement in concrete situations. Thus, in considering Sacred Scripture and tradition, personal experience, and culture in reference to health care, IECs will be contributing to the moral insight of Catholic tradition as a whole.

Footnotes

1. Richard McBrien, *Catholicism,* Winston Press, Minneapolis, MN, April 1980, p. 69.
2. Gregory Baum, *The Teachings of the Second Vatican Council*, The Newman Press, Westminster, MD, 1966. p. 279.
3. W.M. Abbott, *Documents of the Second Vatican Council*, Corpus Books, New York, 1966. pp. 404-405.
4. B. Haring, *Encyclopedia of Bioethics*, Vol.V, p. 1431.
5. *Hospital Progress*, Vol. LIX, May 1976, p. 59.
6. T. Shannon, ed., *Bioethics*, Paulist Press, Ramsey, NJ, 1981. p. 207.
7. Ibid., p. 210.
8. "In Defense of Values," The Catholic Health Association of the United States, St. Louis, 1984.
9. *Hospital Progress*, Vol. LIX, May 1976, p. 44. Also note Keefe's response.
10. Ibid., p. 56.

11. Ibid., p. 55.
12. *Ethical and Religious Directives for Catholic Health Facilities*, United States Catholic Conference, Washington, DC, 1971, 1975. p. 4; also *Health and Health Care: A Pastoral Letter of the American Bishops*, USCC, Washington, DC, 1981. p. 13.
13. Catholic Theological Society of America Report, *Hospital Progress*, Vol. LIV, May 1976, p. 49.
14. *Directives*, p. 1.
15. *Hospital Progress*, Vol. LIX, May 1976, p. 59.
16. Ibid., p. 59.
17. Ibid., p. 59.
18. "In Defense of Values."
19. H. Walgrave, *Unfolding Revelation*, Westminster, Philadelphia, 1972. p. 390.
20. *Directives* p. 4.

■ Workshop Exercises

1. Provide each committee member with a copy of the *Directives*.
2. Have each person write two positive and two negative impressions of the *Directives*. In small groups they should discuss their reasons for responding the way they did.
3. Each person should give examples of the implications of the *Directives* for his or her activities within the institution.

chapter five

Corporate Decision Making:
Five Key Players

Having assessed the impact of religious perspective and role of the *Directives* in ethical decision making, we can now consider the specific roles that various individuals or groups play in achieving moral insight and direction in a Catholic health facility. Depending on their areas of expertise and responsibility, the administration, medical staff, nursing staff, professional theologian/ethicist, as well and the local bishop play significant roles in shaping the institution's ethical character. Ethical insight is achieved in the community through dialogue. Competing interests must be recognized. Sometimes an individual's interests will be challenged by the facility's needs and priorities, while at other times the institution's apparent interests will be called into question by individuals. These conflicts of interest provide grist for the mill of ethical reflection.

Without the healthy tension that the interface of various professional perspectives generates, ethical considerations can often become narrowly focused. The practical consequences of such narrowness can be chilling. For example, a physician who single-mindedly invokes an idiosyncratic ethical vision might run afoul of institutional guidelines, not to mention the standards of his or her own profession. An administrator who implements policies without reference to the medical staff's moral sensibilities runs the risk of alienating an influential constituency. Thus certain key groups and individuals must cooperate in developing a health care institution's ethical character.

Consequently an institutional ethics committee (IEC) should draw on these groups' expertise either directly through securing their representation on the IEC itself or indirectly through instituting effective channels of communication with them. We shall consider five key players: the administration, the medical staff, the nursing staff, the theologian/ethicist, and the local bishop. The practical success of an IEC depends in no small way on its ability to obtain and orchestrate information from these critical sources.

The Administrator

Health care administrators are as directly involved with ethical questions as medical personnel. This may not have been the case in the past, but today it is unquestionably true, although it may not always be recognized. As Dr. Dena Seiden has noted:

> Our society sustains the myth that physicians, and occasionally
> nurses, make life and death decisions for us and control the degree

> of health and sickness. The role of the health care administration is seen as adjunct: balancing the budget, dealing with labor strikes, involving and placating both the local community and the Board of Trustees. In fact, those roles began to change twenty years ago and are now invalid. Physicians and nurses still make immediate decisions on patient care that have implications for life and death [i.e., ethical implications]. But who gets care, when, where, how much, of what quality, and with what technology is, for the most part, no longer determined by clinical personnel. Rather, it is determined by administrators in individual [health care facilities].[1]

Thus, health care administrators today have a very direct responsibility for making decisions of immense ethical significance. They also bear responsibility for their institution's ethical character as a whole.

The administrator has three principal functions in the area of ethical decision making: education, coordination, and implementation. An IEC's effectiveness depends largely on an administrator's willingness and ability to carry out these three tasks.

Education

The administrator's primary duty in education is self-education. One can hardly expect to educate others in the absence of pertinent information and appropriate skills.

Beyond self-education, however, the administrator must educate the institution as a whole by constantly highlighting the significance of ethical concerns. Further, the administrator must concretely display interest in ethical matters by supporting educational programming in ethics for the entire staff. Strong support for the formation and continuing education of an IEC is another obvious means of demonstrating concern for the facility's ethical character.

Finally, in a Roman Catholic facility, the administrator is responsible for educating personnel in the religious and ethical values that guide health care delivery in the Roman Catholic tradition, while at the same time spelling out the practical implications of those values.

Coordination

The administrator should assume responsibility for coordinating ethical reflection within the facility. He or she should strive to create bridges, both internally and externally. Internally, the administration should gather various constituencies (medical staff, nursing staff, housekeeping, etc.) and create a framework for ethical reflection. Creation of an IEC is probably the most practical approach. Beyond the health facility, the administration should seek ways and means of involving the local community and ensuring the appropriate involvement of the local bishop and other religious leaders.

Implementation

Ethical reflection should lead to policy formulation that reflects the fruits of dialogue concerning specific situations. The administrator's responsibility, in cooperation with the board of trustees, is to shape and implement ethically informed policies that flow from an IEC's practical experience and moral reflection.

The Medical Staff

Administrators assuming a more active role in ethically sensitive matters has not diminished the medical staff's involvement. Indeed, the contemporary understanding of medical practice has increased involvement: "Medicine is more than a scientific response to a pathological condition. Because its function is being interpreted more and more in terms of the well-being of the total person, medicine has begun to take into account nonmedical factors, including the values of patients."[2]

In dealing with patients' values, medical staffs inevitably confront ethical dilemmas. Thus staff members play a key role in articulating a health facility's ethical character since they have direct access to ethically charged situations. They are also schooled in the scientific complexities that often cause these situations. In short, the members of the medical staff bring their scientific background and practical experience to bear on ethical issues under consideration by an IEC.

Nursing Staff

The development of IECs has tended to support a parallel development in professional nursing. In recent years nurses have been charting a more independent course. They no longer view themselves as mere assistants to physicians who exercise complete authority and expect unquestioning compliance to medical orders. Nurses have begun to recognize and emphasize their own obligation to exercise some degree of "authority to make clinical judgments and to involve themselves in clinical decisions."[3]

Catherine Murphy describes the independent role of nursing in stating that:

> ...the focus of medicine [is] the nature and degree of pathologic functioning in illness, while the focus of nursing [is] the patient's response to the health problem and the nursing needs which arise from such responses. In other words, physicians diagnose and treat patients' diseases; nurses diagnose and treat patients' responses to health problems which may include responses to disease or medical treatment.[4]

The distinction between the roles of nurse and physician sometimes leads to tension. As Murphy points out, "Physicians use scientific criteria in deciding on choice of treatment while nurses use other types of criteria such as the patient's quality of life and ability to function, cope or adapt in light of the disease and treatment."[5]

Given their divergent criteria for making judgments, nurses sometimes question the ethical propriety of physicians' decisions, and vice versa. Although the contemporary understanding of the nurse's role has given rise to some tension, it has also helped clarify what unique perspectives the nurse can bring to a discussion of ethical issues. Five areas of involvement heighten nurses' awareness of ethical issues and qualify them as particularly helpful participants in the discussion of ethical dilemmas in health care:

1. The nurse is in a position to monitor the patient's quality of life. Quality of life considerations are at the heart of many contemporary ethical debates.
2. Through the nurse's frequent interaction with both patient and family, he or she is in a unique position to help judge whether or not the benefit of medical treatment is proportionate to the burden that the patient will endure.
3. At times the nurse facilitates the patient's involvement in decisions affecting treatment modalities by serving as an advocate of patient autonomy when the patient or guardian have reservations concerning a particular course of treatment. The ethical overtones of such situations are self evident.
4. The nurse is in a position to appreciate the dynamics of the total situation (family relationships, spiritual needs, personal preferences, etc.), since he or she is largely responsible for the overall coordination of the patient's care.
5. Because of insights generated from close and constant contact with patients and family, nurses are drawing attention to ethical dimensions of health care in several areas, e.g., inadequate staffing, lack of equipment, and lack of policies regarding patient care or rights.

Murphy suggests using an IEC to help deal with the ethical dilemmas that nurses are facing today:

> How does a nurse humanely blow the whistle on unsafe institutional practices, unethical practices of other health professionals or honest harm-benefit ratio conflicts with regard to treatment?...Answers are not clear, but it is likely that an ethics committee, where the nurse's input was valued, would be a preferable course.[6]

Thus, nurses can both serve and be served by an IEC.

The Theologian/Ethicist

The theologian serves the IEC by helping to coordinate the sources of moral insight mentioned in previous chapters, i.e., Sacred Scripture and tradition, personal experience, and contemporary culture. As Cardinal Ratzinger has noted, the theologian fosters "...the understanding of the moral demands of the gospel in the particular conditions of his day [personal experience and cultural] and so serves the formation of conscience. In this way he [sic] serves also the development, purification and deepening of the moral [tradition] of the church."[7]

A theologian can contribute to ethical decision making within health care in several ways. For example, the theologian can provide background on Catholic tradition, particularly the historical development of the Church's moral teaching.

It is essential, however, that theologians who work with IECs possess more than a firm grasp of Catholic tradition; they should be more than historians. In other words, the theologian should be familiar with current theological developments and be capable of relating them to the tradition in an intelligible way to the nonprofessional. In selecting a theologian, an IEC must find a person who is comfortable with relating theory to practice and the contemporary context to traditional principles.

In seeking theological resources, the IEC should avoid confusing the roles of the clergy and the theologian. Although most clergy do have background in theology, they are not necessarily professional theologians. It is both unfair to the clergy and unwise for the IEC to assume that clergypersons possess the type of theological expertise that IEC deliberations often demand.

The Bishop

A Catholic hospital represents one dimension of the Church's ministry in a particular locality. As such, it participates in the Church's total ministry, for which the local bishop bears ultimate responsibility. Consequently the bishop plays an integral role in a Catholic health care institution. As noted in Chapter Four, the bishops represent the Church's teaching authority in ethical and religious matters as they find expression in health care delivery. The bishops' specific contribution to health care reflects the general concerns of their pastoral office.

For example, "the bishops should present Christian doctrine in a manner adapted to the needs of the times, that is to say, in a manner that will respond to the difficulties and questions by which people are especially burdened and troubled."[8] It is no exaggeration to say that persons are especially troubled and burdened by the ethical dilemmas inherent in contemporary health care delivery. Thus, the bishop can be expected to encourage the development of doctrine actively in health care areas.

In their pastoral letter on health and health care, the American bishops indicated their determination to respond to current needs:

> At the diocesan level, we intend to demonstrate our commitment to health care by strengthening and adapting those diocesan structures that are involved in the care and maintenance of health. Through our diocesan coordinators of health affairs, for example, we will continue the fruitful dialogue and collaboration that has existed with Catholic health care facilities, with Catholic health care professionals, and with community and state officials within our dioceses.[9]

35

Through this promised dialogue and collaboration, the bishops intend to tap into health care professionals' experience to better understand how Catholic tradition may speak in a contemporary cultural context.

The bishop also plays the role of educator in the public arena. It is his responsibilty to articulate clearly the Church's positions in health care theology and ethics. IEC members have a duty to study the bishop's public statements.

IECs can be valuable resources for the bishop. He can hardly be expected to monitor the health care ethics in his diocese on a day-to-day basis. Even if he could, it is unlikely that he would have the technical expertise to interpret specific medical-moral situations.

Thus the bishop will probably find it helpful at times to turn to an IEC, which could martial the facts and provide necessary background material for his consideration. Moreover, an IEC could alert the bishop to health care developments that might demand his attention.

A relationship between IECs and the local bishop should be maintained, perhaps through the office of the diocesan coordinator of health affairs. This will help guarantee that both the bishop and the IEC have the necessary information to fulfill their respective roles. A smooth working relationship between the two will inevitably improve the quality and ethical tone of health care delivery.

Summary

Various individuals or groups play particular roles in achieving moral insight and direction in a health care facility. The administration, medical and nursing staffs, the professional theologian, and the bishop all contribute unique perspectives to the complex process of developing an institution's ethical character. Forthright dialogue rooted in mutual respect is central to the IEC's task.

Footnotes

1. Dena Seiden, "Diminishing Resources, Critical Choices," *Commonweal*, March 8, 1985, p. 137.
2. L. Weber, *Hospital Progress*, January 1976, p. 68.
3. C. Murphy, *Journal of Law, Medicine, and Healthcare*, Sept. 1984, p. 174.
4. Ibid.
5. Ibid.
6. Ibid.
7. Cardinal Joseph Ratzinger, "Bishops, Theologians and Morality," *Origins*, Vol. 13, No. 40 (March 15, 1984), p. 665.
8. W.M. Abbott, *Documents of the Second Vatican Council*, Corpus Books, New York, 1966, p. 405.
9. *Health and Health Care: A Pastoral Letter of the American Bishops*, United States Catholic Conference, Washington, DC, 1981, p. 9.

chapter six

How to Form the Committee and Educate the Institutional Community

Since different health care facilities have various needs and exhibit different characteristics (e.g., size, location, patient population), the following suggestions for setting up an institutional ethics committee (IEC) will be more or less applicable, depending upon the situation. In our experience, however, six steps typically precede the IEC's formation.

Forming the Committee

First, the need for some type of forum for discussing the increasingly complex nature of ethical health care issues is recognized by an individual or a specific group, e.g., the nursing staff in a long term care facility. The concerned individual or group brings the question to the administrator who initiates a broader dialogue within the institution, drawing on the insights and experiences of key department heads and interested staff.

Given the widespread discussion on IECs today, the group usually focuses on the possibility of setting up such a committee. They discuss an IEC's potential impact and its advantages and disadvantages. Often some resistance to the idea of an IEC develops and the need for a more detailed analysis of the situation rapidly surfaces. Consequently a task force is created to study the advisability of forming an IEC, the second typical step in its development.

The third and fourth steps are the responsibility of the task force. Initially the task force studies existing literature and contacts other institutions that have already formed an IEC. Building on others' experience, they can save time and avoid pitfalls. Task force members then assess the information in light of their institution's needs and resources. At this point they make a recommendation to the central administration—usually a positive recommendation in today's climate. If a positive recommendation is accepted, the task force moves on to the fourth and fifth preliminary steps: working out the description of the IEC's function(s) as well as criteria for selecting members and finally preparing an institution-wide educational program on the IEC.

Since the entire institution will be touched by the IEC's workings, all hospital personnel must be well informed about the background, goals, and functions of the committee before it is formally constituted. The IEC is directed toward improving the quality of the decision-making process throughout the facility, so its workings should be given high visibility and the administrator's support should be seen as unequivocal.

Educational initiatives designed to convey a basic understanding of the IEC as well as strong administrative support may take the shape of special programs for employees, coverage in the in-house publications, and video-taped presentations on the IEC's nature and function. A solid preliminary program will have the double benefit of helping to avoid misunderstandings and fostering increased interest and a willingness to participate.

In the final preliminary step, the task force develops a list of potential candidates for the committee. They interview these candidates and make recommendations to the chief executive officer (CEO), who appoints the committee and names the chairperson. The CEO may also choose to augment the list of candidates presented by the task force, especially if, for instance, a layperson from the local community were to be on the committee.

On completion of the preliminary steps and the appointment of the committee, the stage is set for the IEC's initial formation. The IEC's first responsibility is, as noted in Chapter Two, self education and team building. (See page 9.)

As the committee begins to gel, members will feel the need for more in-depth education. Various consultants may be required to provide background on a variety of issues. For example, the committee might find it helpful to call on experts in such areas as ethics, theology, law, strategic planning, birth/reproductive technologies, and patients' rights in its attempts to deal with such issues as policy making, abortion legislation, concerns regarding euthanasia, church teaching, theological developments, genetic counseling, informed consent, confidentiality, and allocation of resources.

The committee will also have to deal with the issue of evaluation. Ongoing evaluation is essential for committee education and development; however, this important procedure is often neglected by ethics committees. At least two methods of evaluation are required: the committee must (1) develop a method of evaluating itself and (2) devise a method of outside evaluation by the hospital staff. Assessments should be made of the actual policies designed by the committee and the *effects* on and the *effectiveness for* the community. Preferably, evaluations should be made every six months, especially for the two years. Ideally the entire process will help to ensure that the policies do not become static and unattainable by placing unrealistic demands upon the community.

The foregoing steps for forming an IEC should be repeated periodically as new members are added. Care must be taken to orient new members thoroughly to the committee workings and to maintain and increase the other members' understanding of ethical issues.

Educating the Institutional Community

Continuing education, whether formal or informal, is vital to the committee's success. Formal education consists of credit courses, seminars, workshops, and other planned programs. Informal education includes small group discussions, "town hall" types of open forums, information in institutional newspapers, and the institutional "grapevine." Committee members must continually motivate other members and the facility's personnel to participate in continuing education programs.

Motivation is particularly important in recruiting physicians to serve on various committees or to participate in continuing education programs. Personnel who attend the meetings and continuing education programs do so on company time, while the physicians do not. In fact, physicians, who are often in business for themselves, actually can lose money by participating, since they are not reimbursed for lost time. Recognition thus must be given to all committee members. Nonfinancial means of recognition could include official credit for attending continuing education and committee activities, citations for service, etc. Recognizing those who participate can be a powerful motivator.

Formal Strategies

Formal strategies for continuing education can include the following:

1. *Formal courses in ethics, morality, and theology given at the institution.* The state of Michigan recently passed legislation stating that physicians must annually complete 50 hours of continuing education to retain their licenses. Four of the hours must be in medical ethics. Many other states are now considering similar legislation. Hospitals could certify such courses, thereby enabling the physician to count this time as partial fulfillment of the 50-hour requirement. Certain workshops and educational sessions held at the facility could similarly be certified.

2. *General orientation of new personnel.* New employees should be thoroughly oriented to the ethical dimensions of patient care. Initial educational sessions could include lectures, group discussions, or audiovisual presentations.

3. *Ongoing in-service education.* Many organizations send personnel to various programs and seminars to update their knowledge in their area of specialization. The same process can be applied to updating employees' knowledge of medical ethics. For instance, organizations such as the Hastings Center and the Catholic Health Association (CHA) sponsor several educational programs in various parts of the United States that consider various ethical issues in nursing, legal, medical, and pastoral care. Thus a facility could send a designated individual to various seminars; he or she in turn could be required to return and offer a similar session on a smaller scale or to write a summary report or article for in-house publication.

4. *Audiovisual presentations.* Videotapes, facilitated by the institution's communications or audiovisual departments, are another effective means for educating staff to particular issues. Audiovisual programs can produce excellent results because they provide the following advantages:

a. They are mobile in terms of timing and setting; they can be taken to different units at various times and can be made to fit the employees' schedule. Night nurses and other staff members often complain that continuing education occurs only during the day; audiovisual presentations can take place on any shift.

b. Seminars, courses, and lectures given at the institution can be either videotaped or audiotaped and made available to those personnel unable to attend the programs.

c. Audiovisuals can be less time consuming and more cost effective than workshops, formal courses, general orientation, and professional development.

Informal Strategies

Learning occurs in diverse ways and at various times. Education, in the "nonschooling" sense, is never limited to the classroom or the lecture hall. Many educational experiences occur incidentally e.g., while at lunch or on the parking lot. Examples of such informal educational opportunities include:

1. *Written materials.* Significant insights regarding the nature, purpose, and underlying mission of the Catholic health care facility.
   a. Hospital manuals on housekeeping, security, and nursing, for instance.
   b. Effective use of bulletin boards to highlight activities occurring within the hospital.
   c. Articles on ethical issues in the hospital newspaper. This could be a regular feature of every hospital newspaper. Likewise, this paper can play a key role in rewarding employees for their participation in continuing education programs by printing acknowledgements.

2. *Open forums.* Many hospital employees complain about the lack of opportunity for discussion. Open forums in which hospital personnel can react to various policies, problems, etc., can be very effective.

3. *Small group discussions.* These will enable the employees to ventilate their feelings in a constructive manner. There are many purposes for informal small group meetings. They include values clarification exercises, transactional analysis, biofeedback, yoga and forms of transcendental meditation. Informal small group activities can aid in hospital communication.

4. *Social functions.* Wherever people congregate there are opportunities for learning experiences. Through picnics, sports teams, as well as unit and departmental parties, individuals have a chance to get together.

The above does not exhaust the possibilities of informal continuing education strategies. Hospital personnel should be alert to take advantage of these many learning activities.

━━━chapter seven

Approaches to
Ethical Decision Making

Even a cursory review of the functions of the institutional ethics committee (IEC), as outlined in Chapter One, reveals the decision-making role an IEC can expect to play in a health care facility, especially in the areas of policy development, consultation, and case review. Thus the IEC needs some practical guidance in the area of ethical decision making. This chapter is designed to meet that need. After reviewing four common approaches to ethical decision making, we shall draw on some of their respective strengths to offer an integrative model for use by IECs in achieving balanced, ethically informed insights.

As background to our discussion of particular approaches to ethical decision making, we shall briefly consider the notion of ethics in general, since each approach represents a specific way of moving general ethical theory into the concrete, day-to-day experience of persons and institutions.

Ethics

So what is ethics, and how is it relevant to the workings of an IEC in reaching decisions that will affect the entire institution and everyone related to it?

Ethics is one of those "weasel" words that is capable of many twistings and turnings. Everyone seems to know what ethics is—until they are asked to define it.

Dictionaries offer a very limited understanding of ethics. Most define ethics as the discipline that deals with what is good and bad and with moral duty and obligation. These definitions may be technically correct, but they are too general to be of much help to anyone interested in actually *doing* ethics. What is good? How is it determined? Who decides?

Sometimes ethics is also described as a set of guidelines that, if followed carefully, will always lead to good choices and correct behavior. Ethics is viewed as a body of prescriptions and prohibitions, e.g., the *Ethical Principles of the American Medical Association*. This type of "code ethics," although very useful in certain contexts, is too restrictive. It does not do justice to the essence of the ethical enterprise as a whole, which far outstrips concern for a list of regulatory principles.

Ethics aims at developing a reasoning process or method for deciding what *ought* to be done in the face of ambiguous choices, i.e., in the face of alternate ways of acting that exhibit real inconsistency and are logically incompatible in some sense. In other words, ethics devises methods of thinking about human behavior whereby the consequences of that behavior can be evaluated as relatively good or evil and can be judged right or wrong in a particular setting. There are several methods of ethical decision making and for each method, several variations usually exist. Before describing the method we are suggesting that IECs use, we explore a few of the more common approaches to ethical decision making. In this way we hope to familiarize the reader with some of the vocabulary and background of the method we are proposing.

Teleological Model

The term *teleological* comes from the Greek word *telos* which means "end" or "goal." Thus the teleological approach understands ethics in terms of the goal or end of human existence and the means to attain it. God, or in some interpretations nature, directs humankind toward a preestablished goal, and ideally, ethical action reflects that goal. This comprehensive goal or ultimate end unites separate acts into a pattern of meaning that guides one in making moral choices. One first determines what is the ultimate end and then directs individual choices toward the realization of that end. Through either divine revelation, as set down in the Scripture, or reflection on the essential nature of human beings, we uncover eternal laws that govern human action in the world.

When applied to decision making within a health care facility, the teleological approach would call for a decision-making process that would be rooted in the institution's goals. Policy decisions would be considered in light of their capacity to achieve these stated goals. For example, the decision to form an IEC could be understood in light of the teleological approach. A

Figure 1: Teleological Model

1. Perceive the problem

2. List alternatives in light of the facility's goals.

3. For each alternative,

   Assign a value or degree of completion to the goal achieved:
   - a. + + +
   - b. – – –
   - c. +   +
   - d. –   –
   - Etc.

4. Select the alternative(s) with the highest value for the self-realization of patients and staff.

---

nursing home administrator might recognize some serious moral issues in the institution that are not being addressed. The administrator might deal with the issues by administrative fiat, but she recognizes that a stated institutional goal of her institution calls for broad consultation in decision making. Therefore, the administrator decides to set up an IEC to consider the issues at hand.

Figure 1 suggests a teleological approach to decision making.

Formalistic Model

The second type of ethics is formalistic or so-called deontological ethics. The formalistic approach understands ethical life primarily in terms of laws, duties, and obligations. Formalism is not a complete rejection of the teleological approach, but it does have a different emphasis.

The formalist's actions are dictated by ethical principle. Principles and not goals are paramount in analyzing the propriety of an activity. Physicians

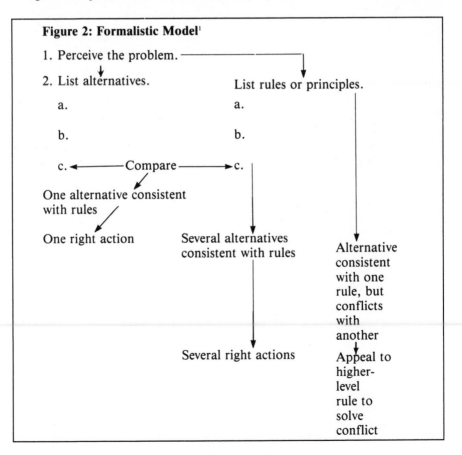

Figure 2: Formalistic Model[1]

1. Perceive the problem.

2. List alternatives.   List rules or principles.

    a.   a.

    b.   b.

    c. ◄———Compare———► c.

One alternative consistent with rules

One right action   Several alternatives consistent with rules   Alternative consistent with one rule, but conflicts with another

Several right actions   Appeal to higher-level rule to solve conflict or nurses who are formalist, for instance, may refrain from participating in direct abortion because they view direct abortion as a violation of the moral principle of respect for life.

According to the formalist approach, the rightness of an act flows from the person's intention to do what is right in principle. Thus formalist physicians who refuse to participate in direct abortion do so, not because of the consequences or the nature of the act itself are wrong, but because they would not be fulfilling their duty to uphold a certain principle.

A formalist asks the following kinds of questions: What are the necessary features of an ethically good life? What makes an ethical life possible? The formalist insists that acting in conformity with an ethical principle (doing one's duty) is *the* essential feature of an ethically good life. The formalist sees no final purpose or goal within nature. An act is considered ethical because a person does it out of duty.

In terms of a dying patient, for example, some physicians might see their primary duty as preserving a person's biological life at all costs whereas others might perceive it as allowing the person to die with dignity. This may lead to a conflict of duty, and it is difficult to know which principle has priority over another based on formalistic criteria. In this context, however, we are not interested in criticizing any single theory. We are simply presenting various approaches to ethical decision making as background to the approach we suggest for IECs.

Figure 2 represents the formalistic or deontological approach to decision making.

Utilitarian Model

Several forms of utilitarianism exist but in general it focuses on the consequences of an action and determines the good act on the basis of an analysis of consequences. Utilitarianism is based on calculating the greatest good for the greatest number of persons. Thus acts that result in the greatest possible good for the most persons in a given situation are judged to be good actions.

Utilitarians contend that an act is good if it leads to an increase of pleasure over pain for a majority in the community. The interests of individuals may be sacrificed to benefit the community as a whole. For example, fetal research and experimentation that could lead to better health care and prevention of disease among children would be morally justifiable because the consequence is positive. This seeking of the general good is the meaning of morality, according to the utilitarian.

Figure 3 outlines the utilitarian approach to decision making.

The following case illustrates the utilitarian approach: Patient confidentiality had become an increasingly apparent ethical problem in a large hospital. Physicians, nurses, and other staff members had been discussing confidential cases during lunch and at coffee breaks. The problem was

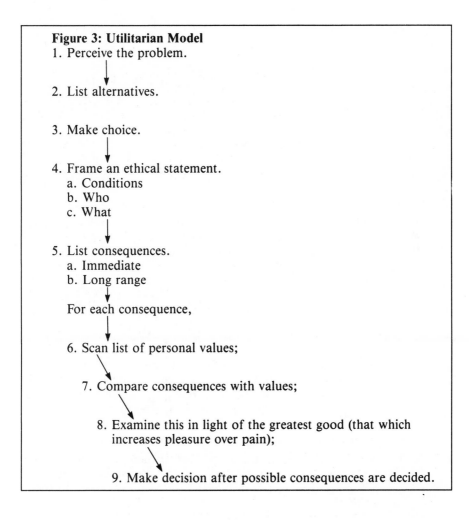

Figure 3: Utilitarian Model
1. Perceive the problem.

2. List alternatives.

3. Make choice.

4. Frame an ethical statement.
   a. Conditions
   b. Who
   c. What

5. List consequences.
   a. Immediate
   b. Long range

For each consequence,

6. Scan list of personal values;

7. Compare consequences with values;

8. Examine this in light of the greatest good (that which increases pleasure over pain);

9. Make decision after possible consequences are decided.

brought to the attention of the IEC, which decided it would be necessary to develop strategies and policies for dealing with the situation.

The committee framed a policy that stated: Since all persons have a right to privacy, staff should not discuss confidential patient information beyond the context of immediate health care delivery. Since the committee was using a utilitarian approach, it listed the consequences of its proposed policy. Then the committee members compared the consequences with the value of the patient's right to confidentiality, and since the consequences were found to be desirable, the policy seemed to be good. More good was achieved for more persons when confidentiality was respected rather than ignored. Thus, since the consequences of the proposed policy supported the greatest good for the most persons, the policy was accepted.

Personalistic Model

A fourth approach to ethics and decision making is personalism. This is the most difficult to explain because it is composed of various strains of thought; thus it is more complex than the other models. We should once again emphasize that these descriptions of various approaches to decision making are merely illustrative; they are not meant to be detailed, and much more could be said.

The personalistic model is primarily concerned with the individual or personal development of each employee and patient. Thus it is oriented toward the individual; its basic focus is the total development of each individual within the community. This approach rests on four assumptions about the human person:

1. Persons are unique. They exhibit original ways of thinking, behaving, appreciating, feeling, etc. Human beings are not puppets on an assembly line; each is characterized by uniqueness and originality that must be respected.

2. Persons are relational beings. They are called in the very depths of their being to be in relationship with others. The "I" is defined by the "Thou." In other words, persons find a large measure of meaning in life through social relationships, particularly those with intimate others (family, friends).

3. Persons are unified. This means that distinctions between body and soul and between mind and spirit, which have pervaded health care in the past, need to be reexamined. For example, human bodies are not accessories. They are not merely something persons have—like the goods they possess. Gabriel Marcel expresses the radical unity of the human person by saying that the person is incarnate spirit.

4. Persons are transcendent beings. Human beings are not merely physical-temporal beings; each person has eternal significance and worth. Figure 4 represents the dynamics of the personalistic approach to decision making.

Using the personalist approach in policy making, the IEC would be concerned with the development of each person within the facility. Policies flowing from this approach would emphasize positive steps to enhance relationships within the institution, especially staff relationships with patients or residents.

Policies developed by the IEC would acknowledge the patient's right to be involved in treatment decisions. The medical staff would be viewed as clinical resource persons who aid patients in decision making. The personalist model would rule out any form of paternalism. Thus policies would support patient autonomy by fostering recognition that patients are unique, relational, unified, and transcendent persons who are, whenever possible, responsible for decisions affecting their medical treatment.

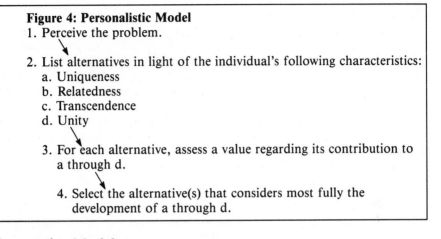

Figure 4: Personalistic Model
1. Perceive the problem.

2. List alternatives in light of the individual's following characteristics:
   a. Uniqueness
   b. Relatedness
   c. Transcendence
   d. Unity

3. For each alternative, assess a value regarding its contribution to a through d.

4. Select the alternative(s) that considers most fully the development of a through d.

Integrative Model

Having provided some background on various approaches to decision making, we now present an approach that we find well suited for use by IECs. If an IEC decides to adopt this approach to decision making, certain steps must be taken in preparation within the health care facility, including:

1. The administration establishes goals that are consistent with the nature and purpose of a Catholic health care facility or, in other-than-Catholic institutions, goals that are consistent with the owners' values. Since these goals will heavily influence the content and direction of the decision-making process, they must be clearly articulated and made available to the entire facility. In this way, the foundations of corporate policy are made clear.
2. The goals are prioritized, since they cannot all be achieved simultaneously. The same value judgments involved in setting goals are generally present in setting priorities.
3. The IEC establishes goals and priorities according to institutional goals.
4. The IEC establishes and defines the committee's goals for an entire year. This provides members with a long-range perspective, which is essential.

If the foregoing steps are neglected, the following approach to decision making may well break down. With these presuppositions in mind, the integrative model is presented in nine steps:

1. Perception of Problem

The committee members must be aware of the complexity of problems. As William James once said, "A problem to be a problem must *be* a problem." Many minute issues will be brought before the committee; the IEC must not become a narrowly focused problem-solving committee. It should stick to the big picture by concentrating on major issues with far-reaching implications. Thus the committee must identify and prioritize issues.

Having perceived a significant issue or problem, the committee must gather data. Speculation cannot replace careful data collection, even though it can be a very time-consuming task. Once the significant facts have been ascertained, the committee is prepared to begin its deliberations.

2. Identification of Alternatives

As simplistic as it may sound, it is important to remember that policy decisions are reliable if they are based on several alternatives. Koontz and O'Donnell write: "If there seems to be only one way of doing a thing, that way is probably wrong."[2]

Alternatives are not always mutually exclusive. Ethical decision making often operates in gray areas. Thus an effective IEC will tolerate differences, for the consideration of conflicting viewpoints often leads to the most tenable policy decisions.[3] Administrative harmony is derived through a consideration of conflict. The members of the IEC should not hesitate to entertain viewpoints different from their own; this will aid in the decision-making process.

3. Evaluation of Alternatives

Since not all alternatives are equally important, the IEC must identify the most relevant ones. Then each significant alternative is evaluated in light of the facility's goal. This is the teleological aspect of the integrative model. Some alternatives can be eliminated because they are inconsistent with institutional goals or objectives.

Alternatives should not be jettisoned simply because they are unpopular or difficult; however, this does happen. One author has pointed out that "often decisions are made not because they further the achievement of the goal, but rather for the convenience of physicians or for the convenience of the institution."[4] An optimal decision often requires courage, since it may be difficult to implement.

4. Consideration of Ethical Principles

After identifying and weighing the relevant alternatives against the institution's goals, the IEC proceeds to examine and weigh the value of each alternative in terms of universal ethical principles. This is the formalistic aspect of the process.

For example, one of the facility's goals may be to serve the community. Imagine that a particular facility is the only health care institution within one hundred miles of a large farming community, and several people in the community think the institution should offer abortion on demand. They believe the community needs an abortion clinic. Some medical staff members believe that the establishment of a clinic is in keeping with the goal of service to the community. Many formalists would rule it out, however, on the grounds that it violates the universal moral principle of respect for life.

5. Evaluation of Ethical Principles

How are universal moral principles known? And once they are known, how are they evaluated? In a Catholic health care facility, these principles are known and evaluated according to the three sources of moral insight discussed in Chapter Four: Sacred Scripture and tradition, personal experience, and culture. These key sources of ethical insight must be considered when trying to reach an informed decision.

6. Consideration of Short-term and Long-term Consequences

The IEC must now ask two questions: What are the short-term consequences of this policy? and What are the long-term consequences? Some alternatives can be discarded because they are inappropriate. In sifting out the short- and long-term consequences of a policy decision, IEC members are using both the utilitarian and the personalistic aspects of the decision-making model. Each consequence of the policy decision should be identified (utilitarian aspect) with regard to the needs of patients, personnel, families, and the community (personalistic aspect).

7. Examination of Consequences

IEC members then can examine the long-term and short-term consequences in light of the facility's goal(s). At times a short-term effect may have to be sacrificed because of its long-term consequence. A policy that merely meets an immediate need may be deceiving since it may turn out to be a long-term disaster. For instance, procedures in x-ray laboratories may facilitate the number of patients treated, but in the long term they may have harmful effects on the employees by exposing them to excessive pressure.

8. Select the Alternative

At this stage of the decision-making process, IEC members should be able to choose the best alternative with regard to the following: the goal(s) of the hospital, the nature of the moral principle(s), the short-term and long-term consequences, and the impact on persons involved. The best alternative can now be expressed in a policy statement. The IEC develops a draft of the policy and the committee members and the administration review it. Personnel who will be substantially affected should be consulted *before* implementation. Revisions, additions, and deletions are made before implementation. In principle, there should be no surprises.

9. Implementation of Decision

Peter Drucker notes three questions to be asked before implementing a policy decision: (1) Who has to know about the decision? (2) What actions have to be taken to carry it out? and (3) Who has to take the actions?[5] IEC members need to consider these questions carefully, since, if approved, the policies they recommend will have to be carried out by other persons.

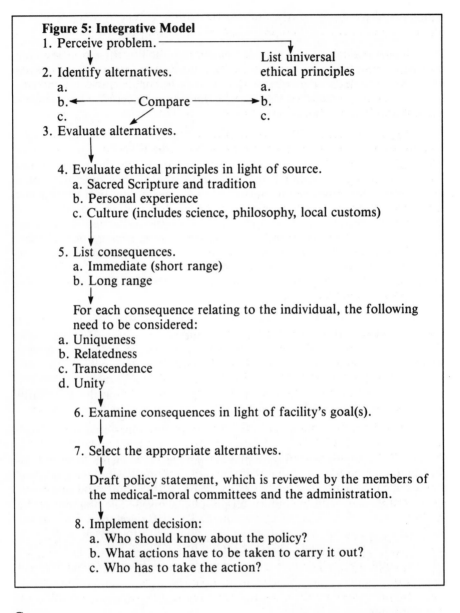

Figure 5: Integrative Model

1. Perceive problem.

List universal ethical principles

2. Identify alternatives.
   a.
   b. ← Compare → b.
   c.
   a.
   b.
   c.

3. Evaluate alternatives.

4. Evaluate ethical principles in light of source.
   a. Sacred Scripture and tradition
   b. Personal experience
   c. Culture (includes science, philosophy, local customs)

5. List consequences.
   a. Immediate (short range)
   b. Long range

For each consequence relating to the individual, the following need to be considered:
a. Uniqueness
b. Relatedness
c. Transcendence
d. Unity

6. Examine consequences in light of facility's goal(s).

7. Select the appropriate alternatives.

Draft policy statement, which is reviewed by the members of the medical-moral committees and the administration.

8. Implement decision:
   a. Who should know about the policy?
   b. What actions have to be taken to carry it out?
   c. Who has to take the action?

Case

It is brought to the attention of the IEC members in a nursing home that patients in the final stages of the dying process who experience cardiac standstill are resuscitated, even though this simply delays death and extends suffering. In the view of many nursing and medical staff, such resuscitation seems unnecessary and overly burdensome for the patient. Thus, the chairperson of the IEC appoints a subcommittee to gather data regarding the problem.

It becomes clear that many physicians are in fact ordering the resuscitation of patients where the benefits are both medically and ethically questionable. After extensive discussion of the issue in the regular monthly meeting, the IEC reaches a consensus: the nursing home needs a policy and guidelines regarding code alerts and related do-not-resuscitate orders.

The alternatives are listed, ranging from patient and family participation in decisions not to resuscitate to decisions made exclusively by the physician. The IEC evaluates the alternate styles of decision making in light of ethical principles. Ethically speaking, the patient has the right to make such decisions. When the patient cannot make such a decision, the next of kin or a duly appointed surrogate should make the decision in consultation with the physician. Either the patient or the patient's representative, may choose to forego excessively burdensome treatment to prolong the dying process, particularly if no realistic possibility of recovery or hope of benefit from the treatment exists. So there are various alternatives regarding decisions not to resuscitate: the patient may decide, the next of kin or a surrogate may sometimes decide, or the physician may decide.

After weighing the alternatives in light of ethical principles governing treatment decisions, the IEC formulates a policy that allows for patients and families to be the principal decision makers in the life-death situations. The physician assists the family by providing medical data. The policy also includes a procedure whereby the physician would indicate on the patient's chart that no code call is to be made in the event of cardiac arrest. The family must request a "no code" in writing.

The IEC then examines both the short-term and long-term consequences of this policy. The facility's legal counsel assists in determining the policy's legality. In the final analysis, the policy is found to be in keeping with the institution's long-term goal(s), since the policy recognizes patients as being transcendent and also recognizes that physical life is not an all-embracing consideration. The continuance of physical life should not be the sole consideration.

The policy is then drafted and reviewed by the committee members, the administration, and other affected parties. An educational program is developed to help implement the policy. The program explicitly explains the reasons for the policy and explicates the procedures to be followed. Finally, the IEC appoints a special subcommittee to examine the effects of the policy on the community.

The integrative approach thus has allowed the IEC members to serve as architects of a healing community in which policies respect the dignity of persons. The IEC has served to harmonize the goals of the individual and the institution.

Footnotes

1. This model is adapted from Howard Brody, *Introduction to Ethical Decisions in Medicine*, Michigan State University Press, East Lansing, MI, 1975, p. A-3.
2. Harold Koontz and Cyril O'Donnell, *Principles of Management: An Analysis of Management Function*, McGraw Hill Book Co., New York, 1972, p. 174.
3. See, for example, Francesca Lumpp, "Ethical Decision-Making," in *Ethical Issues in Nursing Proceedings*, Catholic Hospital Association, St. Louis, MO, 1976, pp. 31-34.
4. Ibid., p. 32.
5. Peter F. Drucker, *Management: Tasks, Responsibilities, Practices,* Harper & Row Publishers, Inc., New York, 1973, pp. 476-477.
6. This exercise was adapted from a similar case in Howard Brody, *Ethical Decisions in Medicine*, Little Brown and Co., Boston, MA, 1976, p. 39.

Workshop Exercise

1. Decision-Making Study Case No. 1

Part I

Mr. Y has had a biopsy taken of an enlarged lymph node. The biopsy report indicates a malignant lymphoma. A more thorough physical examination has turned up a mass in the patient's abdomen. All indications point to its being of lymphatic origin and also malignant. Mr. Y repeatedly asks for the biopsy report, and Dr. Z refuses to tell him the diagnosis and its implications.

On several occasions while awaiting the report, Mr. Y has told Nurse X that if the biopsy showed cancer, he would not want to live. Mr. Y is becoming increasingly agitated because of evasive answers from his physician, Dr. Z. Mr. Y's physical condition is worsening daily. Despite medications, Mr. Y is unable to sleep. On a particularly sleepless night when Nurse X is on duty, Mr. Y calls her and asks: "Please tell me the truth, the report shows that I have cancer, doesn't it?" What should be Nurse X's response?[6]

Decision making is selecting a course of action from alternatives. How should Nurse X make her decision?

Individually, have the participants:

1. List possible alternatives open to Nurse X.
2. Evaluate the alternatives in light of moral principles and values.
3. Evaluate the consequences (immediate and long range) of each alternative.
4. Select the best alternative.
5. Explain specifically why your decision was made from the best alternative.

Part II

Have the participants in small groups discuss their decision and the reasons they chose that as the best alternative.

Part III

In groups of four, have the participants share their best alternative and their reasons why. Next, have the participants do the following:

1. Evaluate the consequences of each participant's decision:
   a. Both immediate and long range
   b. In light of effects on individual patients and nursing staff
   c. With regard to the facility's goal(s) and purpose
2. Have the group come to a consensus as to the best alternative for both the patient and the institution.
3. Have the participants formulate a policy statement for the facility regarding future dilemmas such as the case explicated.

53

4. Have the participants design a plan for implementing the following:
   a. Who in the facility needs to know of the policy?
   b. What actions have to be taken to implement the policy effectively?
   c. Who has to take the action? In the large group have each group share its policy decisions.

━━━━chapter eight

Scenario: St. Lynda Sets Up An Institutional Ethics Committee

A scenario is an Italian word referring to an outline or a synopsis of a play or an opera; the scenario includes various acts of the play and lists the players' entrances and exits. In the motion picture industry a scenario is invaluable to the director, since it outlines the plot of the movie, showing its development scene by scene.

In this chapter, the scenario is a fictionalized account of how a particular institution went about forming an Institutional Ethics Committee. The plot unfolds scene by scene, with a few instructions for the major players in the drama. We stress that the following account is completely fictional and does not represent an actual institution. We should also note that this is but one scenario that is by no means exclusive.

St. Lynda Hospital is a 500-bed, general health care facility approximately 20 minutes from the downtown area of a large city. The hospital was founded in 1929 and at that time served primarily middle- and upper-income people. Throughout the years the hospital maintained an outstanding reputation for excellence, and many prominent physicians sought to join its staff.

Today, however, the hospital is in the midst of a rapidly deteriorating neighborhood. Some staff physicians have moved their practice to the more affluent suburbs. The hospital now serves mostly the poor and indigent. Because of the burgeoning costs of health care delivery, recession, and an inflationary economy, the hospital was forced to close its obstetrical unit. Inpatient admissions total approximately 17,000, with an average daily census of 450 to 475. The occupancy remains fairly constant at 80 to 85 percent. Besides the departments ordinarily found in a health care facility of this size, St. Lynda has a kidney center and a clinic with various outpatient services. It is also a teaching hospital with a nursing school and residency program.

The CEO, Mrs. Newman, a competent administrator with many years of experience, is highly respected by the staff. She is noted for her commitment to the consultative management approach, especially management by objectives. Consequently, in weekly administrative staff meetings and department head meetings the staff establishes and evaluates objectives in light of the hospital's general goals.

Recently, the staff has brought several ethical problems to Mrs. Newman's attention. For instance, the outpatient clinic's director has been concerned about the number of physicians encouraging their patients to have sterilizations. In some cases the physicians have reportedly encouraged abortions. There is also mounting pressure for the hospital to be more flexible in its sterilization policy.

55

Moreover, the head of the department of medicine has noticed that physicians permit what he considers an excessive use of advanced technology to delay the deaths of certain patients. Also, the director of nursing services has gotten numerous complaints regarding abuses of informed consent and the quality of physician-patient relationships.

When ethical problems such as these arose in the past, Mrs. Newman usually consulted with the chaplain, the department involved, or with the physician to resolve the difficulty. The chaplain, Rev. Smith, is a conscientious individual who possesses a good working knowledge of the *Directives* but he has little background in ethics. Thus he often feels quite inadequate when Mrs. Newman asks him to offer an opinion.

At a convention of Catholic chaplains, Rev. Smith shares some of the difficulties he has experienced in dealing with ethical problems at St. Lynda. The other chaplains sympathize; they are having similar problems. One mentions a new approach to dealing with ethical issues that his hospital has recently adopted; he calls it an institutional ethics committee (IEC).

Rev. Smith shares the idea of an IEC with Mrs. Newman, who is immediately interested. She has the hospital librarian research the literature on ethics committees. Then she contacts other Catholic hospitals to find out if they have a committee to deal with ethical issues and how to go about forming one. Mrs. Newman decides to move slowly but as expeditiously as possible.

Rev. Smith contacts a number of moral theologians, asking if they have been involved in the development of such a committee. To his surprise, several have, and they express a willingness to lend a hand at St. Lynda.

Both Mrs. Newman and Rev. Smith are excited about the possibility of forming an IEC, so they arrange for a resource person, George Jones, PhD, to visit the hospital and give the staff a lecture on the potential benefits of such a committee. After the meeting, several complaints arise. Some staff members do not think that the hospital has enough significant problems to warrant the development of such a committee. Others say that far too many committees exist already. Some physicians believe that an IEC might undermine the physician-patient relationship.

Although the staff does not unanimously accept the idea, several do commit themselves to exploring the feasibility of an IEC at St. Lynda. A task force is set up which begins its discussion by considering the role and function(s) of an IEC in an institution such as their own. They agree that an IEC could serve as a center of reflection and expertise to deal with the ethical issues becoming increasingly prominent in their daily lives. They see the IEC as a forum where ethical issues could be identified and discussed with the potential for developing policies and guidelines to provide a framework through which others could make appropriate, concrete, ethical decisions.

The next important item for discussion is how to get the committee started. Mr. Anderson, the associate administrator, suggests appointing committee members; after this, an orientation session might occur. Rev. Smith, however, disagrees, saying that a hospital-wide educational program should come before appointing a committee, since the IEC would have much more support if everyone understood why it was being formed. Dr. Jones agrees.

Mrs. Newman asks Dr. Jones to meet with Rev. Smith, herself, the medical staff president, and the director.

Meanwhile, the educational program has begun. Dr. Jones starts by giving a brief talk concerning the rationale for the committee to the various groups within the hospital. The sessions will be videotaped for future use at orientation programs and for those unable to attend the sessions.

The task force now must appoint IEC members. Mr. Anderson and Mrs. Newman meet with the various department heads to discuss possible candidates. They confer with the chief of the medical staff, the director of nursing services, the social welfare department, the department of psychiatry and so on. The task force wants to be careful to give the committee an ecumenical perspective; it also wants to have a balance of men and women on the committee.

After much evaluation, the following members are decided on: the Catholic associate administrator will represent the hospital administration; a local bank vice-president, who is a Baptist, will represent the board of trustees; and a humanist neurosurgeon will represent the surgical staff. Likewise, the committee would include a female Methodist obstetrician, a specialist in internal medicine who is a Hindu, a female social worker who is a Presbyterian, a Catholic lawyer, a Catholic nurse from the intensive care unit, and a Jewish psychiatrist. Rev. Smith will represent the pastoral care department.

The day for the first meeting finally arrives. A secretary is appointed to keep the minutes. Mr. Anderson initiates the discussion by asking three questions:

1. What is our purpose in being here?
2. What do you see as the goals for the IEC?
3. How should they be implemented?

The questions stimulate a great deal of discussion, but some obvious communication problems become apparent.

When Mr. Anderson and Mrs. Newman meet after the meeting, they both agree that the members need some training in group process, since they noted some defensiveness within the group. Some of the nurses felt intimidated by the physicians, while other committee members felt obliged constantly to turn attention to the Church's teaching on any matter that came up for discussion. Thus many blocking mechanisms had surfaced during the first meeting.

The second meeting focuses largely on the interpersonal problems at the first meeting. Questions for the agenda include: How do you feel prepared to serve on this committee, and how do you feel unprepared? Where are the obstacles to your successful participation on the committee? The questions bring out some interesting issues. The non-Catholics say that they do not feel prepared to deal with ethical issues that are mainly Catholic in nature. Most members suggest that they do not feel prepared at all. The group decides that they need a training session to prepare them for participation in the decision-making process. Mr. Anderson and Mrs. Newman are delighted at the results of the meeting, since it is important for the committee members themselves to identify their needs. This allows the members to be fully responsible for the IEC's functioning and generates a sense of ownership.

At the third meeting, Dr. Jones is asked to help plan the training program. The committee members believe that they need more specific information from Dr. Jones, as well as more small group work. Dr. Jones presents the following program outline to the committee members:

Session I: The Catholic hospital as a healing community. This includes a brief overview of the Catholic hospital's historical development and an examination of a Catholic facility's distinct characteristics.

Session II: A discussion of ethical decision making.

Session III: A discussion of the need and value of the *Ethical and Religious Directives*

Session IV: An introduction to various models of ethical decision making that can be used in a hospital setting.

Session V: A presentation of the IEC's role and function.

Time becomes a real problem. A single monthly meeting is simply not enough to move the committee through its formative stages, so the committee members decide that they will meet for seven consecutive Wednesdays from 1:00 to 2:30 PM. Each Wednesday there will be a presentation for 45 minutes followed by a coffee break. Then the members will break into smaller groups using either discussion questions or case studies pertinent to the topic. At the end of the seven weeks, Dr. Jones meets with the committee to evaluate the sessions. The committee members have found that the sessions were very profitable.

Some key issues surfaced during the training sessions; for instance, the problem of physicians not being as open as they might be in the presence of nurses. Physicians also are reluctant to discuss certain medical-moral issues because such a discussion might intimidate their colleagues. The IEC decides that although this is serious, it is not the time to confront it. Mr. Anderson suggests that if the problem does not resolve itself in time, he will personally take positive steps to rectify the situation by discussing it with the individuals involved.

As part of the training session the committee members have studied the philosophy of St. Lynda Hospital. At the next meeting, Mr. Anderson suggests that the committee develop its goals and objectives for the coming year in light of this philosophy and what they learned during the initial formation period. The members agree, and each acknowledges that he or she is now ready to investigate some of the ethical problems in the hospital community. So, in preparation for the next meeting, they decide to attempt to prioritize the problems presently existing.

The next monthly meeting proves to be very controversial. The IEC members bring up such issues as informed consent, the hospital's sterilization policy, responsible parenthood counseling in the clinic, and racial discrimination in the emergency room. As the various issues emerge, some members become very defensive, especially if the issue concerns them directly. By the time the meeting adjourns, it borders on a shouting match.

Several problems emerge from the meeting, especially the intimidation of nurses by physicians. Mr. Anderson and Mrs. Newman come to the conclusion that it is time to deal with this issue. Mr. Anderson decides to meet with each physician and nurse on the committee privately. In his meetings with the physicians, a number of issues are clarified. The physicians view themselves as objective scientists, and they resent the criticism of nonmedical personnel. They are also businesspersons who lose money each time they attend committee meetings. The hospital personnel on the committee are using hospital time and thus are paid; the physicians are not.

Mr. Anderson spends a great deal of time reflecting on ways to overcome these difficulties. So at the next meeting, two subcommittees are formed. The first consists of physicians from the existing committee and from the hospital's medical staff; the second would consist of paramedical personnel. The purpose of the subcommittees is to discuss crucial issues, such as communication between physicians and nonmedical personnel. The members of each subcommittee would suggest policies for improving conditions. These policies then are brought to the IEC for comment and revision.

Within two months, conditions improve. The physicians have their subcommittee in which they can discuss key issues without criticizing their colleagues in front of other personnel. The paramedical members have the same opportunity and freedom within their subcommittee. Eventually Mr. Anderson realizes that other subcommittees are needed.

The members of both subcommittees find that the issues of informed consent and the physician-patient relationship are their top priorities. At the next monthly meeting, Mr. Anderson suggests that the issue of informed consent needs further research. The physicians will research the topic from their point of view, especially in regard to what information they are giving patients and their effect on the patient and the family. A staff nurse is asked to do the same from the nurses' perspective. The social worker will research the patient's rights in this matter, the legal advisor will research the legal implications for the hospital. Rev. Smith is to consider the theological literature, the *Directives*, and any Church teachings on the matter.

At the next meeting each person reports on his or her study regarding informed consent. The physicians report on the various methods being used to inform patients regarding medical and surgical procedures and the difficulty in explaining these procedures to patients, because of fear of a malpractice suit. The nurses feel limited in explaining procedures to patients, especially in the absence of the physician, who is often excessively busy. The nurses also feel hindered, since they are legally restrained from explaining various procedures to patients. The social worker emphasizes the hospital's philosophy which includes the concern for each patient as unique and deserving of respect. The lawyer explains the legal implications of informed consent. They all agree that a policy should be written to ensure patients' rights to be informed.

The legal counsel further elaborates on the legal implications. He reports on court interpretations of informed consent adopted by the Supreme Court of California and Rhode Island. He discusses the famed *Canterbury vs. Spence* decision in Washington, DC, where it was concluded that the patient must be informed of all material risks. The materiality of the risk is determined primarily by the significance a reasonable lay person would attach to such a risk. Thus the witness of the medical community is not the determining factor. The lawyer continues by suggesting that a physician may be held liable if he or she fails to disclose pertinent information.

Rev. Smith then presents his findings. He has investigated the work of important theologians on the topic of informed consent. Likewise, he has referred to Section One of the *Directives* which deals with this issue.

After much discussion, a consensus is reached and the committee agrees to draft a policy regarding informed consent. Two committee members volunteer to work with Mr. Anderson in drafting a tentative policy based on the committee's discussion for approval at the next meeting.

At the next meeting, a policy is approved and a plan for implementation is designed. Some key questions emerge, however, for instance, "Who should know of the policy?" and "What actions have to be taken to carry it out?" The committee members decide that all hospital employees should be informed of the policy, especially those directly involved with patient care. Special meetings would be held with the chief of medical affairs and the director of nursing services. Their advice is critical to the effective implementation of the proposed policy.

Someone suggests that a special subcommittee be formed to provide ongoing assistance in implementing the policy and in reviewing its effects on the hospital community. This subcommittee would be chaired by a physician who serves on the IEC. This subcommittee would also be responsible for ongoing educational programs in this area.

After the first year, the hospital community began to respond more positively to the IEC. Mr. Anderson continued to send a resume of topics discussed and problems resolved to the board of trustees, the administrator, and the bishop.

After two years, the committee was able to work through most of its initial blocking mechanisms successfully. The physicians and nurses felt freer to engage in dialogue regarding hospital issues. The medical and paramedical subcommittees have been retained to give each group the freedom they need to prioritize issues and discuss ethical dilemmas in their respective areas of expertise.

Figure 1 shows the organization structure of the IEC after two years.

After two years, the committee faced the problem of replacement and subsequent training of new committee members. The tenure for committee members is two years, and most members decide to stay on the committee for another two years. One of the physicians, however, is moving his practice elsewhere and must be replaced.

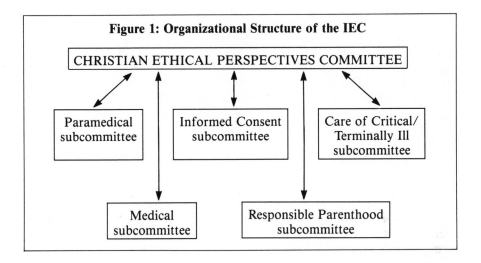

Figure 1: Organizational Structure of the IEC

Mr. Anderson also feels that he ought to resign as chairperson. Another person on the administrative team accepts the chairperson's position. She agrees to meet with the committee for a certain time to observe its operation. She is also willing to receive further preparation in ethics.

The problems at St. Lynda are far from being eradicated. Yet the hospital now has an instrument that can creatively deal with ethical issues. The committee members have also learned how to train hospital personnel to encourage the effective implementation of policies. The IEC has helped unify the hospital community. This has necessitated greater communication among the various departments. St. Lynda is far from perfect, but the development of an ethics committee has greatly improved the quality of the decision making and greatly enhanced communication and understanding within the institution.

━━━━━━━━━━chapter nine
The Committee Meeting: Nuts and Bolts

Are two heads better than one? Generally speaking, the answer is, "Yes." It has been demonstrated that "the results of a group are distinctively superior to the results of the average member and are equal to those of the best members."[1] Social psychologists constantly remind us that, all things being equal, groups usually make better, more fully informed decisions. The National Aeronautics and Space Administration (NASA) has developed an exercise that underscores the strengths of group decision making.

The so-called NASA Exercise offers participants an opportunity to experience the advantages of group interaction. Participants are asked as individuals to rank what they would need if they were marooned on the moon. Then they are asked to do the same in a group. Having conducted this simulated survival game with several government and industry management groups, James Owens concluded that "the group score is almost always (in 95 percent of the cases) better, often dramatically so, than the average of the individual scores."[2]

Institutional ethics committees (IECs) are an attempt to capitalize on the strengths of group decision making. As N. Fost and R. Cranford have noted, "Diverse viewpoints often lead to better decisions, (and) ethics committees, according to this view, may be more likely than individual(s) to arrive at decisions that, in retrospect, will withstand ethical scrutiny and legal challenge."[3]

But how do groups make decisions? How do persons act and react in groups? The following section is designed as a general introduction to the group dynamics, especially the role of the group leader (IEC chairperson). It is an attempt to provide very practical information on the conduct and content of committee meetings.[4]

The Chairperson's Role

Mention a committee meeting to most persons, and they will tell you how frustrating and unproductive they are and how much time they waste. In fact, a camel has often been described as a horse designed by a committee. Many think that ineffectiveness is synonymous with meetings.

Groups are not ineffective, but often the members in them are. As a chairperson, you will be called on to attend and to lead meetings. You can make these meetings very productive if you plan and execute them properly. The three primary parts of meetings are preparation, the meeting, and follow-up. This chapter deals with meetings in an order-of-event method.

Preparation

Careful planning is as important to a successful meeting as its management. Certain issues need to be addressed *before* the meeting is held.

Meetings should have a real purpose. They may be held for various reasons, but they should always have a rationale for meeting that is more than "We always meet on the third Tuesday of the month." This rationale should be stated in terms of goals.

Topics vs. Goals

A common mistake among group leaders is to confuse goals with topics. A topic may be a project's status, the departmental budget, the new piece of equipment, or an employee problem. Identifying the topic does not identify the goal. For instance, if the topic is a problem concerning the employees, the meeting's goal may be to identify the cause of the problem and decide on some working solutions, to follow up on some solutions suggested at an earlier meeting, or to decide how to prevent the problem from recurring. Similarly, if a topic is the departmental budget, the goal may be to give a status report to those concerned, to find new ways to cut the budget, or to discuss the ways the last budget cut has affected employee morale.

The meeting's goal should be identified before any other decisions are made. In fact, identifying the goal will facilitate these other decisions. If, for example, a goal cannot be identified, then a meeting will be a waste of time, money, and resources for all who may have attended. Identifying a goal gives you a reason to have a meeting.

Reasons for Meetings

One of the best reasons to have a meeting is a direct result of modern technology and the specialization that has subsequently occurred in an effort to keep pace with it. It is not only impractical but improbable that any one person within an institution can solve major ethical problems without the advice or consultation of other departmental employees. In deciding whether or not an issue should be brought to the IEC, the chairperson should consider the following questions:[5]

1. How important is the quality of the decision? (How many persons will it affect?)
2. Do you possess enough information and expertise to make a high-quality decision?
3. To what degree do others, taken as a group, possess information needed to make the decision?
4. If you make the decision alone, will it be accepted and carried out by others?
5. Will others be motivated to carry out the decision or policy?
6. To what extent are involved persons likely to be in disagreement over the solution to the problem?

7. How important to effective implementation is acceptance of or commitment to the decision?

These questions will help you determine if you need a committee to make a decision.

Types of Meetings

Many reasons exist to have a meeting other than decision making. A list with a brief explanation of each type of meeting follows.

1. *Informational.* These meetings are held to disseminate facts, which may consist of:
   - Decisions made on policy and procedure
   - Information about hospital events
   - Data on new product usage
   - Educational/training material used to expand the knowledge and/or skills of employees' performance
   - Other in-service information
2. *Planning.* The purpose of this meeting is to develop long-range plans or to formulate strategy to deal with anticipated problems. These meetings are concerned with the future.
3. *Problem Solving and Decision Making.* Plans also are made in these meetings, but they are formulated to deal with current problems. The decisions should generate action within a short period. The focus is on daily activity rather than future goals. A decision is made on how to deal with a problem that has occurred or is occurring.
4. *Follow-up.* These conferences are held to ensure the progress of plans made in problem-solving and decision-making or planning meetings. Progress reports are provided and feedback is obtained on organizational performance. These meetings provide the forum for formal evaluation.

After deciding on the type of meeting that will best meet the objective, you can move on to the next phase of preparation.

State the Goal

The goal has been identified, a need for the meeting has been established, and the type of meeting has been chosen. The goal should be written down, and a specific outcome should be stated. In other words, how will you know when your goal has been reached? Is it possible to attain your goal in one meeting, or will it necessitate holding several meetings? Once these questions have been answered, you can determine the particulars of the meeting.

Proper Facilities

The availability of proper facilities is necessary before a meeting can be held. Proper facilities are defined as any appropriate area that will allow the meeting members to be free from distractions and comfortable. The area and furniture should also enhance communication by being well lit and well ventilated and arranged to permit everyone to contribute easily.

Included in proper facilities is the need to make proper equipment and visual aids available to participants who may wish to use them.

Develop an Agenda

Before the meeting, develop an agenda based on the goal(s) you have set. Keep the following factors in mind when deciding on agenda items:

- The type of meeting to be held
- The degree of controversy of each item
- The size of the group
- The talkativeness of the group members
- The length of time the group usually takes to complete the goal if similar situations have occurred in the past.

Include only as many items on the agenda as you think the group can handle in a reasonable period.

Identify Necessary Information

Using the agenda as a guide, try to determine if you can make the meeting more productive by preparing certain types of information in advance. If, for example, you plan to refer to a particular article, make copies of the article and summarize the pertinent parts to prevent wasting time during a meeting while someone reads a report.

Notify the Participants

You are finally ready to notify the meeting members of their desired attendance. Any oral notice should definitely be followed by a written notification. This notice should include:

- Location
- Time (beginning and ending)
- Date (ideally two weeks, but at least one week advance notice)
- Topic identification
- Goals and objectives of the meeting
- An agenda (most important items first)
- Any preparations you expect the members to make before the meeting, including any materials you want them to bring
- A copy of any information you want them to be familiar with before the meeting
- Some method of determining whether or not the individuals will attend, and whether it is acceptable to send a representative

It may be necessary to remind the participants of the date, time, location, purpose, and objectives of the meeting a day or two before the meeting.

Conducting the Meeting

Content

As the meeting leader, you are responsible to guide the group members toward the goal. The following rules are followed by all successful meeting leaders.

1. *Start on time.* You have already notified the members of the starting time; it is their responsibility to arrive on time. If you wait for late-comers, you are indirectly suggesting that the starting time was not important, and assumptions may be made that other items on the agenda may not be important either. Besides, it is frustrating for members who do arrive on time to have to wait and waste their time. Starting on time rewards those who arrive on time, sets a precedent for your future meetings, and allows the meeting to develop more productively.

   If you begin a meeting late, you begin with frustrated members and members who assume this meeting really is not important. None of these persons will be able to contribute much to attaining the goal. If this is the case, little reason may exist to hold the meeting at all.

2. *Review the priorities.* This can be accomplished by reviewing the agenda. In most cases the agenda is composed of a list of items in order of importance. The exception to this is when one of the items may elicit an emotional response that would be more difficult to handle than other items. This exceptional item may be scheduled for a later time despite its importance. The exception to this is when the group leader is particularly good at handling difficult situations. This type of leader may want to take advantage of the freshness of a meeting by tackling the hardest issue first.

3. *Stick to the agenda.* Control of a group is lost when a leader allows committee members to bring up issues not listed on the agenda or to use an agenda item as a jumping off point for other issues. When control is lost, the meeting's purpose is lost. Without a purpose, no meeting should be held.

   If new items are introduced, they can be assigned to a list of agenda items for a future meeting. To maintain credibility, you are responsible for ensuring that those items are dealt with at some reasonably near date. If the meeting ends early, the new items can be dealt with in the remaining time.

   Time is set aside for each agenda item based on an educated guess. Discussing new, nonscheduled items will infringe in most cases on the allotted time reserved for another item. Although some committee members will be concerned about being confined to discussing specific topics at specific times, research has shown that more members will be upset if all the agenda items are not covered as intended. They lose their sense of closure for the meeting's purpose and will

67

become frustrated and perhaps angry, after only one or two such incidents, particularly if they have prepared information that they intended to share on a specific item that was then postponed or dropped.

4. *Assign responsibilities and target dates for task accomplishment.* If the purpose of the meeting is problem solving or decision making, then the solutions and decisions need to be implemented. Assigning implementation to specific members ensures its accomplishment. Assigning a target date for completion ensures timely completion. Besides solving problems, it gives the committee members a sense of accomplishment. A change in attitude can then be developed in those who had previously viewed meetings as unproductive and a waste of their time.

5. *Summarize decisions.* Toward the end of the meeting, you should take a few moments to go back over the decisions that were made. This not only reinforces a sense of agreement within the group, but gives the participants a chance to clear up any misinterpretations.

6. *Close the meeting at or before the agreed time.* If the committee members are asked to stay "just a few more minutes," it shows either a lack of proper planning or a lack of good meeting leadership. If the meeting was held to the agenda, then the items not covered will be the last ones on the list and in most cases can be put off until the next meeting. If the meetings regularly run over, too many items are put on the agenda or insufficient time allowed for problem solving. In either case, corrections should be made so that this becomes the exception rather than the rule.

    Most meetings can accomplish their goals in one to two hours. It is difficult to maintain interest after two hours. If more time is necessary for decision making or problem solving, split the goals into minor objectives. Not only will you now have the time to complete the agenda, but you will also be giving the members a sense of completion after each meeting.

    It is important to obtain agreement on decisions, but this agreement is difficult to maintain if members stop caring about your meeting's purpose and start worrying about how they will not be able to complete the work they had scheduled during these "few moments" you have asked them to stay. In other words, you lose more than you gain when asking members to stay beyond a predetermined time.

7. *Maintain written records of the meeting.* Minutes should be taken during the meeting and then distributed to members as soon as possible after the meeting. Minutes provide a source of recall about what happened and what decisions were made, as well as a written reminder for those members who were assigned certain tasks during the meeting. *Caution*: An IEC should guard confidentiality by deleting explicit references to individuals by name.

Process

A group needs to have certain functions attended to if it is to be productive. Without these functions, progress will be slow and goal attainment will be difficult, if not impossible. It is the leader's responsibility to see that the meeting progresses well. The functions previously mentioned are dealt with in detail here so that chairpersons may study and learn from them.

1. *Define the problem.* As soon as the meeting is convened and the agenda distributed, the leader must take time to state the goal and define the problem as clearly as possible. As each problem is solved or each decision made throughout the meeting, the leader is responsible for defining the next problem (issue) on the agenda.

2. *Propose procedure.* The leader also is responsible for identifying the limits of possible procedural solutions. You should not dictate the procedure to be used but should suggest some viable ones. For instance, you might say that only certain resources are available or that a particular time restraint exists. Based on the restraints, you might then suggest that the solution be discussed in part among smaller subcommittees, or you might give each individual a chance to offer a solution. You might also want to ask for procedural solution ideas from the other committee members. A meeting leader should never dominate, but should always lead.

3. *Involve members.* A major function of leaders is to encourage participation of all group members. Leaders can use group involvement to find out if everyone understands, or to obtain a variety of opinions. To increase participation, leaders may have to encourage some members to speak up but also discourage some from speaking so much. After all, if each IEC member was invited because of his or her expertise or ability to contribute, then it is your responsibility to see that each receives that opportunity.

   Those who do not offer their opinion readily may be willing to do so with a little encouragement. Often this can be accomplished by just asking for their opinion. Occasionally you may have to use a bit more encouragement, but always remember the difference between encouraging someone and embarrassing them. A committee member who has been embarrassed will not contribute constructively to the meeting.

4. *Clarify and elaborate.* Often referred to as "gate keeping," this is the committee leader's primary job. Some of the responsibilities of this function include:
   - Controlling the amount of conversation. Limit comments to about two minutes. Meetings are not the proper places for speeches.
   - Controlling the direction of conversation. Limit comments to one idea. Complete each topic before going on to new material.
   - Clarifying all statements made. Without this, the group may move on to another area before they fully understand what was just dis-

cussed. Paraphrasing is a good way to make sure everyone has the same meaning in mind.

- Being a good listener. Be sure you hear what is said, and observe the nonverbal communication as well. Notice if someone is having a hard time "getting a word in" or if they show obvious objections to what another is saying, etc.
- Not making evaluative statements. Your responsibility is to clarify what was being said, not to judge it.

5. *Summarize.* This, too, takes careful listening. In order to summarize, you must be able to restate differences of opinion. You must be able to reflect on what the group has done. This is not a time for your personal opinion. Sometimes you may need to stay out of the discussion altogether and just take notes so that you can give a better summary. Summaries should be made after each major agenda item. Summaries help to:

- Remind the group of decisions that were made.
- Focus the group on the tasks.
- Provide a transition to the next agenda item.
- Prevent misunderstanding of decisions made.

6. *Test consensus.* After summarizing each issue, the leader should ask each person for a brief opinion. This is done only to discover the degree of agreement or disagreement, and not to get everyone to agree. When asking for individual opinions, it is best to ask first those who are least likely to influence others. This prevents "group think," i.e., having less influential individuals pretend to agree with the more powerful people in the group when no such agreement actually exists.

7. *Make assignments and give directions.* It may be obvious who could best carry out a particular task. If it is not, you can then either ask for volunteers or give assignments randomly. Also, set an expected completion date for assignments.

8. *Conclude the meeting.* Before a meeting is adjourned, a final summary should be made about what decisions have been made and who is going to do what by when. No one should leave a meeting without a clear understanding of the decisions made, the actions expected, the persons responsible for implementation, and the timetable. You should also try to end on a positive note; a word of encouragement or appreciation is helpful.

Dealing with Conflict

Being a group leader is a relatively easy task if the meeting has been well planned and all the members contribute positively to goal accomplishment. Careful planning is crucial to a successful meeting, but even with such planning, meetings sometimes fail to reach their goal because of disruptive individuals.

If every group member had the same point of view and no conflict or disagreement ever occurred, the meeting would flow very smoothly. It does seem a waste of time, energy, and money, however, to gather such a group together. There would be no real purpose in the meeting. In such cases it would be more efficient and just as effective to disseminate the information through a memo or report.

Some amount of conflict is a healthy, necessary part of meetings. Such conflict often results in the exploration of new ideas; members are often stimulated to create new alternatives, and the result may be a better solution to the problem. To achieve this end, the group leader needs to know how to deal with disagreements and conflict so that it contributes to the meeting's effectiveness. Without this skill, the conflict may grow and become disruptive.

The leader can deal with such conflict in several ways. Each way is successful when used in the right situation, but each also has its drawbacks when used exclusively.

The five most common ways of dealing with organizational conflict, according to Simpson are:[6]

1. *Denial or withdrawal.* In this approach the group leader often tries to ignore the conflict, refusing to acknowledge it during the meeting or the summaries. This method can be effective if settling the conflict has little to do with the meeting's goal. You must remember, however, that denying a conflict exists may enable you to complete the meeting on time, but it will not alleviate the conflict. Without some attention, the conflict may grow out of proportion or may interfere with other goals.

2. *Suppression or smoothing over.* A meeting leader using this method will play down differences that arise between group members. Although this method is useful if dealing with the differences will not contribute to goal attainment, it is not the best method to employ if they need to be resolved. Remember, suppressing a problem may make it more difficult to solve when it arises again, and it will.

3. *Power or dominance.* Often used to settle differences, power may be manifested through the group leader or through majority dominance. Although power is used frequently, for instance, during elections or other types of voting procedures, problems may arise from its use. The most frequent one is a result of the win-lose situation that must always occur: the majority or the leader wins; all others lose. The losers are frequently the cause of future problems. They may resist accomplishing necessary tasks. They may harbor a grudging resentment that may carry over into the next meeting.

4. *Compromise or negotiation.* This particular method of dealing with conflict is often seen as the most humane, virtuous approach. We seldom study the serious drawbacks of this method. First, with advanced knowledge that compromise will occur, many individuals will inflate their demands, knowing that they will give up a certain

71

portion of them during the bargaining process. Second, if this inflation does not occur, then each individual's desires may be so compromised as to be "undesirable." If this happens, each side may be so dissatisfied with the outcome that there may be little commitment by anyone to carry out the compromised solution.

5. *Integration or collaboration.* Integration is similar to compromise in that individuals change their original expectations. The major difference is that, in integration, these changes are a result of new decisions made by members through increased information made available to them. Each member is encouraged to make data available that impact on the problem or situation, and a group effort is then made to use this data to formulate the best possible decision. Although this appears to be an ideal solution, it is most effective when no constraints of time, money, or resources exists and committee members are willing to make decisions for the common good rather than personal departments or issues.

Dealing with Individual Behaviors

Handling the problems of groups would be easier if leaders did not also have to deal with the problems of individual members. Finding the proper solution to a problem, is often difficult, but it is frequently impossible if disruptive members are permitted to control the meeting and not allow it to progress.

General techniques. Several general methods are available for handling difficult members. According to Mike M. Milstein, the following rules can help improve the committee leader's ability to deal with difficult members.[7]

1. *Listen but do not debate.* By listening to them, you will allow the debating members to feel as if their opinions are respected. Then try to work their comments into the mainstream of the discussion. Through this, dissenting members will often try to focus their energy on working to solve the problem at hand.

2. *Talk privately with members who continually exhibit disruptive behaviors.* Berating a committee member in public will definitely not encourage him or her to work toward problem resolution with the group. It may even worsen the behavior. A private counseling session preserves the individual's dignity, prevents others from being embarrassed from witnessing a public chastisement, and conserves meeting time as well.

3. *Turn negative behaviors into positive contributions.* Some committee members' behavior may be seen as disruptive when they are not intended as such. Some members may not be aware of proper procedure or of the most effective way to accomplish goals at meetings. Setting a good example may solve the problem. If it does not, the leader can try to channel energy into productive procedures by assigning specific meeting tasks to these individuals. Perhaps they could be responsible for summarizing or gate-keeping.

4. *Encourage the group to share the responsibility for handling difficult members*. Negative, disruptive behaviors are more likely to decrease if the other committee members disapprove of them. Group pressure is usually more effective than any single leadership attempt at control. Disruptive members are usually a lot less willing to have the entire group upset with them than they are to have just the leader upset. As a leader, you can take advantage of this and encourage group censorship of the particular disruptive behavior.

Specific Individual Techniques. Sometimes disruptive members must be dealt with on an individual basis that addresses a particular behavior. The following is a list of the most common disruptive behaviors along with suggestions for dealing with these.[8]

1. *Eager beaver traits*. These persons interrupt frequently to give information or to "help clarify" situations. They try so hard to help that they actually make it difficult for others to express an opinion. As soon as someone begins to speak, they interrupt with their "support." *Solution*: Cut across these persons tactfully by questioning others. Thank them for the input, and then suggest that "we put others to work." You may want to assign them the responsibility of summarizing so that they are forced to listen.

2. *Challenger traits*. These persons have a combative personality or may be a "professional heckler." Although they may be normally good natured, they may be upset about something and taking it out on the group. More likely than not, they enjoy being aggressive and deflating others' ego. *Solution*: Keep your own temper firmly in check; do not let the group get excited either. Try to spend your time reaching your goals, not defending yourself. Most of the time the challenges are made to the group leader. Toss them back out to the group; let them handle it. As a last resort, talk to the challenger privately and explain why you see this behavior as unproductive.

3. *Know-it-all traits*. Sometimes the know-it-all is just a show-off, but sometimes she is exceptionally well-informed. Whatever the problem is, she has the definitive answer. *Solution*: Do not be embarrassed or sarcastic...she *may* have the definitive answer and you may need her later on. Slow her down with some difficult questions. Interrupt with "That's an interesting point...now let's see what the group thinks."

4. *Star traits*. The star seeks recognition. Unlike the know-it-all or the eager beaver, the star does not think he has all the answers or can do a better job of leading than you can. He speaks up just for the recognition. He is usually a loud or excessive talker, often with extreme ideas or unusual behavior. He does not try to be humorous, just noticed. He'll talk about everything except the subject. *Solution*: When he stops for a breath, thank him for his contribution, refocus his attention by restating the relevant points, and move on. If he was really off on a tangent, take the blame for it. Say, "Something I said

73

must have led you off the subject. This is what we should be discussing..."

5. *Tongue-tied traits*. This person understands what is happening and is thinking of some good ideas, but lacks the ability to express herself properly. She just cannot put her thoughts into words. *Solution*: She needs help. Do not embarrass her by saying, "What you mean is this ..." Instead, say, "Let me repeat that for the group." Then put the idea in better language. Twist her ideas as little as possible, but have them make sense.

6. *Lost soul traits*. This is the person who comes up with a comment that is obviously incorrect. He may have misunderstood something *or* he may have made the comment just to get sympathetic attention. If this is the case, his comments are usually preceded with "This is probably wrong, but..." or "I don't know if this is what you mean, but..." Even though he knows his comments do not address the issue, he makes them anyhow. What he hopes to gain is sympathy. He wants others to think, "Poor man. Look how hard he tries." *Solution*: If he misunderstood, explain again what may have caused the confusion. If he is trying to gain sympathy, get the meeting back on track by acknowledging the remark but not giving the expected sympathy. Say, "That's one way of looking at it" or "I see your point, but can we reconcile that with the (true situation)?" Encourage him to get attention by coming up with plausible solutions, not by trying to get sympathy.

7. *Devil's advocate traits*. She points out all the reasons why something will not work. She tries to put you on the spot. She may also support an opposite point of view, but not because she believes it. *Solution*: Never take sides. Use her opinions in your summary and ask others what they think of them. Point out that your view is relatively unimportant and that the group's view is what matters. There are times when you must, or should, give a direct answer (e.g., when her comments are leading the group off the track).

8. *Daydreamer traits*. He withdraws from the meeting by acting bored or indifferent. He gazes out the window, doodles, whispers to others, or busies himself with unrelated matters. *Solution*: Your action will depend on what is motivating him. If he is bored, arouse his interest by asking for his opinion. If he is withdrawn because he feels too insecure or timid to participate, encourage him to respond and reward him with praise for doing so. If he is feeling superior, ask him for his view after indicating the respect held for his experience. Do not overdo this.

9. *Fighters' traits*. Usually seen in pairs, these members clash over everything. Even if they agree with the other fighter, they will not admit to it. A single fighter in a group will resort to blocking. She will interfere with the progress of the group by going off on a tangent, citing personal experiences unrelated to the problem, arguing too

much on one point and rejecting ideas without consideration—anything to get someone to fight with her. *Solution*: Emphasize points of agreement between fighters; minimize points of disagreement. Draw their attention to the objectives. Cut across their fighting with direct questions on the topic. With both fighters and blockers, involve others and then draw their attention away from the fighter or blocker. Ask them for positive feedback on points made by others.

10. *Mule traits.* This person just will not budge. He thinks he is right and will not consider anything that might make him change his mind. Although he does some blocking, he does not want to fight with anyone. *Solution*: Throw his view to the group members and have them straighten him out. Tell him time is short, and you will be glad to discuss it with him later. Ask him to acknowledge the group's viewpoint for the moment.

11. *Confessor traits.* She uses the group as a sounding board. She expresses personal feelings about unrelated topics and tries to get the group to solve her personal problems. *Solution*: As a group leader, you are responsible for sticking to the agenda. Do not address the issues she brings up. Say "We can put that issue on a future agenda, but today we need to consider (topic). Do you have any comments on that?" This will let her know that you care enough to consider her problems in the future, but it keeps everyone on track for the meeting.

12. *Competitor traits.* What the competitor really wants is to be the best ...the one with the best ideas, the one who is best at everything. He'll stick to the topic, as long as he knows that everyone else agrees with what he has to say. Unlike the star, who is serious but often goes off the track, the competitor "stays in the race." *Solution*: Recognize the contributions made by the competitor. He will try to come up with a viable solution to problems. But do not allow him to discourage others from contributing. Ask for other opinions. It will encourage him to work toward an even better solution.

13. *Clown traits.* Unlike the star or competitor, the clown is not serious. While a little humor is a good thing, the clown carries it to extremes. He seems always to be joking or horsing around. He disrupts the group's work. *Solution*: Attention is a reinforcement for behavior. Ignore the clown's silliness but pay attention to any positive, serious contribution he might make. Give him a special assignment that may increase his concentration.

Improving Member Behavior

When reviewing the nonfunctional behaviors described, keep in mind that some of these behaviors will be seen in all groups at some time. And when they occur, they may not be disruptive. A little clowning may give group members the relief from serious matters when they need it. A devil's advocate may cause them to think of a better solution. A competitor may stimulate some creative thinking.

Even if these behaviors surface continuously, you still have two options. First, you must take a serious look at your leadership abilities. Are you allowing this behavior to occur or even encouraging it because of your inability to deal with disruptive behavior in meetings? Perhaps you should ask someone else to chair the meetings, or perhaps you should review methods of dealing with the behavior so you are prepared to handle the situation.

Second, keep in mind one of the first things you considered when organizing the meeting: Is the disruptive person a necessary member of the committee? If he is, it is your responsibility to the rest of the group to call the disruptive behavior to his attention. If he is not necessary for goal attainment, the solution is obvious: don't ask him to be a committee member.

As group leader, you are responsible for letting the members know what roles are expected of them. It is also your responsibility to practice your gatekeeping techniques so that you can perform your leadership duties effectively.

Other Group Behaviors

Tension in a meeting is likely to occur for several reasons. If you are moving through the agenda too quickly, members may feel that they are not being given a chance to express their opinions fully. If members of one department sense that they are being asked to sacrifice too much for the institution's good, they will feel tense about it. This feeling may escalate into a conflict among committee members. Tension may also result from a meeting which has lasted too long, a meeting being held at the end of a long day, or one in which members are unable to reach a solution to problems.

These situations can be resolved by organizing the meeting so that it occurs earlier in the day, has fewer agenda items, and allows members to state their opinions freely and to try to solve problems honestly instead of just talking about them. Tension can also be relieved by having a short refreshment break or by using a little humor (not to be confused with sarcasm, which only increases tension).

Hidden agendas. Groups work on two levels. One level is the surface task, i.e., the reason for calling a meeting; the other is the level of individuals' hidden, undisclosed needs and motives. These needs and motives are generally those that members would like to fulfill during the meeting, even though they are not listed on the meeting agenda. These are called hidden agendas. Accomplishing the task at hand is difficult if group members are expending their energy on their hidden agendas.

Many of the disruptive behaviors discussed earlier are the result of a particular individual's hidden agenda. Although each person will need to be handled according to his or her particular behavior, a leader can do some things for groups so that meetings can progress smoothly without hidden agenda interference. Wilson and Kneisl have the following suggestions for for dealing with hidden agendas:[9]

Suggestion	*Rationale*
Look for the presence of hidden agendas.	The group cannot diagnose or solve a problem until its presence is recognized.
Once the presence of hidden agendas has been pinpointed, judge whether or not they should be brought to the surface and rectified.	Sometimes hidden agendas should be left undisturbed if the consequences of bringing them to the group's attention group may be negative, rather than facilitating their work.
Determine whether group members are willing and able to deal with hidden agendas. Suggest that perhaps not all there is to say has been said, but do not force members to self-disclose their hidden agendas.	Self-disclosing hidden agendas may be harmful to group attempts to reach cohesion and may result in the premature ousting of the member with the hidden agenda from the group.
Accept members whose hidden agendas have been revealed, without rejecting or criticizing them.	Hidden agendas are common and legitimate group occurrences. They should be worked on in the same way that group tasks are.
Devote group time to working on the hidden agendas of members.	Hidden agendas impede group progress. The amount of attention given to hidden agendas should be determined by the extent of the effect on group performance.
As a group, evaluate the group's ability to deal with hidden agendas.	Learning better ways of handling agendas more openly will result from evaluation and reduce the need for keeping agendas hidden.

Follow-up

After every meeting, a follow-up is necessary to make sure the group has accomplished the meeting's goal. A systematic follow-up will adhere closely to the following guidelines:

1. *Review the objectives.* Were the goals and objectives of the meeting met? If not, try to determine what caused the failure. Perhaps too many goals or objectives were set. Perhaps too many disruptions

occurred or too much (or too little) was said about them. The list is nearly endless. The point is that you should examine all aspects of the meeting. If you can identify a problem, decide how you can overcome it before the next meeting.

2. *Compare the use of time to the accomplishment of objectives.* Did you schedule enough time for each agenda item? Did you schedule the right amount of agenda items? Was the meeting concluded at the scheduled time? Were the accomplishments worth the members' time and effort?

3. *Prepare and distribute minutes.* Both the group leader and the recorder should go over the minutes and check them for accuracy. Remember, these minutes, after approval by members at the next meeting, become an official record of meeting activities. Minutes should be distributed within two weeks of the meeting, if possible. (The sooner, the better.)

4. *Send out individual action-review sheets.* It is the group leader's responsibility to follow up on plans made in meetings. One very effective way to do this is to send out individual reminders to committee members, listing what that individual agreed to accomplish. Ask for feedback on accomplishments so you will know whether or not a reminder note is necessary.

5. *Distribute committee action-review sheets.* In addition to serving as a reminder of commitments, committee action-review sheets serve as a notice of others' progress. This gives recognition to those completing their tasks and encourages others to get their tasks done.

6. *Send out appreciation and recognition notes.* When the plan is accomplished, a note of recognition to committee members will let them know that their work was appreciated. It encourages them to participate in future committees because they will feel that both the committee and their work was worthwhile.

7. *Schedule unfinished business.* All matters scheduled but not attended to at the meeting should be put on the agenda for the next meeting. Putting it at the top of the agenda indicates that it was important but that time did not allow for it to be addressed. Putting it at the end of the next agenda or leaving it off altogether indicates its lack of importance. If it is that unimportant, perhaps it should never have been included in the first place. When scheduling an agenda, ask yourself how important it is to cover it during a meeting, and where it would be placed on the next agenda if it were not addressed at the scheduled meeting. You can eliminate many unnecessary items this way.

The Meeting's Participants

An effective meeting depends not only on appropriate leadership, but also on the participation of its attendees. When asked to be a meeting participant, keep the following suggestions in mind.

1. *Prepare for the meeting.* Make sure that you understand the meeting's purpose and agenda. Then organize your thoughts and be prepared to offer any information that may be necessary to accomplish the meeting's goals. Prepare any material that may facilitate problem solving.
2. *Participate during the meeting.* Offer any information you have. Question statements or ideas on which you need clarification. Assist in problem solving by offering thoughts and suggestions that will move the meeting in a productive direction.
3. *Be aware of your behavior.* Do not dominate the meeting or participate in any of the dysfunctional behaviors discussed earlier. Be aware of the type of reaction you usually exhibit in meetings. In most cases you will be able to identify with one of the following behaviors:
   - *Work* - preference for task-oriented or problem-solving behavior.
   - *Fight* - expressed as angry responses; may be verbal attack, subtle resistance, or manipulation of group to one's viewpoint.
   - *Pairing* - another person's idea is supported; warmth, commitment, and supportiveness are expressed to another member or to the whole group.
   - *Dependency* - reliance on rules, regulations, and definite structures; dependency on leader or outside authority; expression of personal inadequacy.
   - *Flight* - preference for escape of any kind (withdrawal, joking, daydreaming, irrelevancy of statements, excess personal activity).
4. *Be aware of others' behavior.* If no one is gate-keeping (keeping the meeting on track), do so yourself for the committee's good. Ask for summaries or give them yourself. Study the disruptive behaviors and solutions for handling them and offer to assist the leader if he or she seems unable.
5. *Analyze the meeting.* After the meeting has been adjourned, analyze it. Was it worth your time and effort? If not, how could it have been improved, and what can you do to help it improve? Offer any suggestions to the group leader.

Footnotes

1. Robert B. Zajonc, *Social Psychology: An Experimental Approach*, Brooks/Cole Publishing Co., Belmont, CA, 1969, p. 99.
2. Derived from the *Desert Survival Problem*, developed by J. Clayton Lafferty and Patrick M. Eady, copyrighted by Human Synergistics, 1970.
3. "Guidelines for Ethics Committees in Healthcare Institutions," *Journal of American Medicine*, May 10, 1985, p. 2698.
4. Mike M. Milstein, "Toward More Effective Meetings," *1983 Annual for Facilitators, Trainers, and Consultants*, University Associates.

5. Victor H. Vroom and Phillip W. Yetton, *Leadership and Decision-Making*, University of Pittsburgh Press, Pittsburgh, 1976, p. 421.
6. Donald T. Simpson, "Handling Group and Organizational Conflict," *1977 Annual Handbook for Group Facilitators*, University Associates, pp. 120-122.
7. Mike M. Milstein, "Toward More Effective Meetings," *1983 Annual for Facilitators, Trainers, and Consultants*, University Associates.
8. Developed by Dr. Christine Bruce, Corporate Manager of Education and Development, SCH Health System, Houston.
9. Holly S. Wilson and Carol Kneisl, *Psychiatric Nursing*, Addison-Wesley Publishing Co., Reading, MA, 1979.

chapter ten
Evaluation Guidelines

Definition of Evaluation

1. The measurement of results in relation to stated goals, policies, and action plans
2. The asking and answering of the question: "Are we doing what we said we were going to do?"
3. The building in of procedures for objective self-analysis *at every step* in the process

A significant distinction exists between evaluation and review. Review is that process whereby the institutional ethics committee exercises its right to question an entire process or program.

Questions To Be Considered During Evaluation

- Did we do what we said we would do?
- How do we feel about what we did? Was it worthwhile?
- In what ways could it have been done more effectively?
- How do others feel about what was done?
- How do we feel about the procedures that were followed in carrying out our action plans?
- As a result of what was done, what have we learned about the overall mission and ministry of the institution?

Evaluation takes place at the end. At the end of a project or a program, at the end of the year, we tend to evaluate what has happened. This addresses itself to the questions, "Did we do what we said we would do?"

An evaluator can experiment with many formats. Once an evaluation is completed, the results should be returned to the participants. If the participants know that they will receive the compilation of evaluations they will be more interested in the evaluation itself. It will also demonstrate the leader's concern for his or her group.

Malcolm Knowles gives a listing of questions that we consider necessary for proper evaluation:[1]

- Are the purposes of any proposed evaluation clear and understood by all parties who will be involved?
- Have plans for evaluation been made as part of the program-planning process?

- Have realistic priorities been set that will result in the most important improvements?
- Have all parties who will be affected by evaluation been represented in planning it?
- Have the most efficient and reliable means for getting the desired data been used?
- Are the data being adequately analyzed and the findings being fed back into the planning process?
- Are those from whom data were obtained being kept informed about the findings and the use that is being made of them?

Question Formulation

The purpose of evaluation is to find out if the objectives of a program have been achieved. It is also important to discover if any behavioral change has been initiated by the participants.

The evaluation questions should be stated in such a way that the participants would indicate the benefits, or lack of benefits, of the program.

1. Questions should never be such that they require only yes or no answers.

2. Questions should be open-ended, allowing for personal comments by participants.
   - Poor: Did you find this program helpful?
   - Good: What did you find most helpful about the program? What did you find least helpful about the program?
   Questions such as these help to partialize the program and pinpoint the successes and/or failures.

3. To discover if the program created problems, include questions on the format and process of the program.
   - How effective were the speakers?
   - Were you satisfied with the presentation? Why or why not?
   - How many times did you participate in group discussion? Why or why not?
   - What suggestions do you have for improving this kind of program?

4. Build in questions that will help the participants pinpoint a behavioral change.
   - What will you do differently now that you have been involved in this program?
   - How has this program motivated you to get involved in some activity?
   - How will you personally use the information (knowledge, technique, skills) you have gained from this program?
   - What problems do you presently anticipate as you try to implement the information, etc., you have gained?

- Specifically, what is your present plan for using this training and experience in your local situation?

NOTE-All these questions do not have to be included in one evaluation. They are given as samples and should be adapted to program and participants.

5. Design questions that will force persons to be specific. This is valuable to the programmer, since he or she can get feedback that will be helpful in the future.

Subjective Evaluation Sample

1. What were the ways you saw this experience as being helpful?

2. If it wasn't helpful, how would you rather have spent this time?

3. What were the two most important things that happened to you in this session?

4. If you were to experience this session again, what would you change?

5. In terms of meeting your needs and expectations, how would you rank this session?
   Poor_____ Fair_____ Pretty Good_____ Very Good_____

6. Other comments:

Evaluation

This evaluation is meant to be given to departmental personnel for whom the IEC created and developed policies.

Sample of Evaluation of Discussion Session

1. Were you satisfied with the topic selected for the discussion?
   Very little_____   Moderately_____   Great deal_____
2. To what extent did you feel free to talk about the issues and policy suggestions?
   Very little_____   Moderately_____   Great deal_____
3. How effective do you think this policy and discussion has been?
   Not at all_____   Moderately_____   Very effective_____
4. Did you learn anything from it?
   Nothing_____   Little_____   Very much_____
5. Was there need for more resource material?
   Yes_____   No_____
6. To what extent did you feel you were listened to?
   Not at all_____   Sometimes or moderately_____
   Usually_____   Always_____
7. How would you rank this session in terms of its helpfulness to you?
   Poor_____ Fair_____ Pretty good_____ Very good_____
8. Do you intend to learn more on the topic?
   Yes_____   No_____
   If yes, what resources will you use?
   _____
   _____
   _____

9. Will you do anything differently in your department as a result of this session?   Yes_____ No_____
   If yes, what?_____
   _____
   _____

Footnote

1. Malcolm Knowles, *The Modern Practice of Adult Education: From Pedagogy to Andragogy*, Cambridge Books, Cambridge, MA, November 1980, p. 229.

Appendix I

Resources: Articles

Allen, P.A., et al. Development of an Ethical Committee and Effects on Research Design. *Lancet* 1(82-83):1233-36, May 29, 1982.

Allen, D.F., and Fowler, M.D. Cognitive Moral Development Theory and Moral Decisions in Health Care. *Law, Medicine and Health Care* 10(1):19-23, February 1982.

Annas, G.J. CPR: When the Beat Should Stop. *Hastings Center Report* 12(5):30-31, October 1982.

Annas, G.J., In re Quinlan: Legal Comfort for Doctors. *Hastings Center Report* 6:29-31, 1976.

Annas, G.J. Informed Consent and Review Committees, in *Psychosurgery Debate*, Elliott S. Valenstein, ed. San Francisco: Freeman Press, 1980.

Annas, G.J. The Quinlan Case: Death Decision by Committee. *New Physician* 28(2):53-54, February 1979.

Annas, G.J. Refusing Treatment for Incompetent Patients: Why Quinlan and Saikewicz Cases Agree on Roles of Guardians, Physicians. *New York State Journal of Medicine* 80(5):816-21, April 1980.

Aroskar, M., Anatomy of an Ethical Dilemma: The Theory. *American Journal of Nursing* 80(4):658-63, April 1980.

Bader, Barry, and Burness, Andrew. Ethics: Boards Address Issues Beyond Allocation of Resources. *Trustee* 35:14, October 1982.

Bader, Diana. Medical Moral Committee: Guarding Values in an Ambivalent Society. *Hospital Progress* 63:80, December 1962.

Baron, C.H. Medical Paternalism and the Rule of Law. *American Journal of Law and Medicine* 4(4):337-6 365, Winter 1979.

Basson, M.D. Choosing Among Candidates for Scarce Medical Resources. *Journal of Medicine and Philosophy* 4(3):313-333, September 1979.

Bayley, C. Terminating Treatment: Asking the Right Questions. *Hospital Progress* 61(9):50-53,72, September 1980.

Bayley, C. Clinical Setting Enhances Bioethics Education. *Hospital Progress*, 64(12):50-53, December 1983.

Bayley, C. Who Should Decide? *Legal and Ethical Aspects of Treating Critically and Terminally Ill Patients*, A.E. Doudera, D. Peters, eds., Ann Arbor, AUPHA Press, 1982.

Beresford, H.R. The Quinlan Decision: Problems and Legislative Alternatives. *Annals of Neurology* 2:74-80, 1977.

Biomedical Ethics: A Symposium. *Virginia Law Review* 69:405-561, April 1983.

Breur, H., et al. Role of Ethical Guidance Committees in Clinical Research. *Controlled Clinical Trials* 14: 421, May 1981.

Brodeur, Dennis. Toward a Clear Definition of Ethics Committees. *Linacre Quarterly* 51(3):233, August 1984.

Buchanan, A. Medical Paternalism or Legal Imperialism: Not the Alternatives for Handling Saikewicz-type Cases. *American Journal of Law and Medicine* 5(2): 97-117, Summer 1979.

Buchanan, A.E. The Limits of Proxy Decision-Making for Incompetent Patients. *UCLA Law Review* 29(2): 391-96, 1981.

Campbell, J.D., et al. The Hospital Ethics Committee. *Medical Journal of Australia* 1(4):168, February 1980.

Caplan, A.L. Can Applied Ethics be Effective in Healthcare and Should It Strive to Be? *Ethics* 93:311-319, January 1983.

Capron, A.M. The Quinlan Decision: Shifting the Burden of Decision-Making. *Hastings Center Report* 6:17-19, 1976.

Capron, A.M. A Statutory Definition of the Standards for Determining Death: An Appraisal and a Proposal, in *Biomedical Ethics and the Law*, J.M. Humber and R.E. Almeder, Eds. New York: Plenum Press, 2nd ed., 1979.

Cebik, L.B. The Professional Role and Clinical Education of the Medical Ethicist. *Ethics, Science, and Medicine.* 6(2):115-21, 1979.

Childress, J.F. Who Shall Live When Not All Can Live? in *Contemporary Issues in Bioethics*, T. L. Beauchamp, ed. Encino, CA: Dickenson Publishing Co., 1978.

Cohen, Cynthia. Interdisciplinary Consultation on the Care of the Critically Ill and Dying: The Role of One Hospital Ethics Committee. *Critical Care Medicine.* 10:776, November 1982.

Committee on the Legal and Ethical Aspects of Health Care for Children, Comments and Recommendations on the "Infant Doe" Proposed Regulations. *Law, Medicine and Health Care.* 11(5):203-209, 213. October 1983.

Cranford, R.E. and Doudera, A.E. The Emergence of Institutional Ethics Committees. *Law, Medicine, and Health Care.* February 1984.

Cranford, R.E., et al. Institutional Ethics Committees: Issues of Confidentiality and Immunity. *Law, Medicine, and Health Care.* April 1985.

Curran, W.J. Quality of Life and Treatment Decisions: The Canadian Law Reform Report. *New England Journal of Medicine* 319(5):297-298, February 2, 1984.

Cushing, M. Law for Leaders. "No Code" Orders: Current Developments and the Nursing Director's Role. *Journal of Nursing Administration.* 11(4):22-29, April 1981.

David, P.P. Psychiatric Considerations for the "Right to Pull the Plug." *Illinois Medical Journal* 155(6):380-383, June 1979.

Decision Making for the Incompetent Terminally Ill Patient: A Compromise in a Solution Eliminates a Compromise of Patients' Rights. *Indiana Law Journal.* 325-48, Spring 1982.

Denham, M.J., et al. Work of a District Ethical Committee. *British Medical Journal.* 2(6197):1042, October 1979.

Doudera, A.E. Editorial, Section 504, Handicapped Newborns, and Ethics Committees: An Alternative to the Hotline. *Law, Medicine, and Health Care.* 11(5):200, October 1983.

Editorial: The Decision to Die: Who Makes It? *Lawyers Weekly* 6:596, 1979.

Ethics Committees and Ethicists in Catholic Hospitals. *Hospital Progress.* 64(9):47-56, September 1983.

Esquada, Kathi. Hospital Ethics Committees: Four Case Studies. *Hospital Medical Staff.* November 1978, p. 26.

Fama, A.J. Classification of Critically Ill Patients: A Legal Examination. *Saint Louis University Law Journal.* 24(3):514-553, October 1980.

Farley, Margaret A. Institutional Ethics Committees As Social Justice Advocates. *Health Progress.* 65(10):32, October 1984.

Fish, M.S. Euthanasia: Where Are We? Where Are We Going? *Journal of the Medical Society of New Jersey.* 778(12):812-815, November 1981.

Freedam, Benjamin. One Philosopher's Experience on an Ethics Committee. *Hastings Center Report.* 11:22, February 1981.

Freeman, J.M., and Rogers, M.C. On Death, Dying, and Decisions. *Pediatrics.* 66(4):637-638, October 1980.

Glaser, Jack, (ed.). A Model for Forming a Medical-Moral Committee. *Ethic Notes.* December 1981, Farmington Hills, MI; Sisters of Mercy Health Corp.

Guidelines to Aid Ethical Committees Considering Research in Children: Working Party on Ethics of Research in Children. *British Medical Journal.* 280(6209):229, January 1980.

Guidelines to Ethical Committees Considering Research Involving Children. *Archives of Disease in Childhood.* 55(1):75, January 1980.

Guidelines for Hospital Committees on Biomedical Ethics, Chicago: American Hospital Association, 1984.

Guidi, Doris Jordan, *Hospital Ethics Committees Potential Mediators for Educational and Policy Change.* Dissertation, Fairleigh Dickinson University, 1983.

Gutteridge, F., et al. The Structure and Functioning of Ethical Review Committees. *Social Science and Medicine.* 16(20):1791-800, 1982.

Hamilton, M.P. Role of an Ethicist in the Conduct of Clinical Trials in the U.S. *Controlled Clinical Trials.* (14):411-20, May 1981.

Henry, C. The Ethics of Ethics: Nurses Participation on Ethical Committees. *Nursing Mirror.* 156(24):30, June 15, 1983.

Hirsch, H. Establish Ethics Committees to Minimize Liability, Authority Advises. *Hospital Risk Management.* 3(4):45, April 1981.

Holmes, C. Bioethical Decision-Making: An Approach to Improve the Process. *Medical Care.* 17(11):1131-38, November 1979.

How Can Medical-Moral Committees Function Effectively in Catholic Health Facilities? *Hospital Progress* 64(4):77-73, April 1983.

John Paul II, Pope. A Patient is a Person. *Medical Service* 39(2):13, 15, 17 passim, February 1982.

Keenan, Carol. Ethics Committees: Trend for Troubling Times, *The Hospital Medical Staff.* 12(6):2, June 1983.

87

Leenan, H.J.J. The Selection of Patients in the Event of a Scarcity of Medical Facilities—An Unavoidable Dilemma. *International Journal of Medicine and Law*. 1(2):161-180, Autumn 1979.

Lestz, P. A Committee to Decide the Quality of Life. *American Journal of Nursing*. 77(5):862-866, May 1977.

Levin, D.L., and Levin, N.R. DNR, An Objectionable Form of Euthanasia. *University of Cincinnati Law Review*. 49:567-579, 1980.

Levine, Carol. Hospital Ethics Committees: A Guarded Prognosis. *Hastings Center Report*. 8:25, March 1977.

Levine, M.D., et al. Ethical Rounds in a Children's Medical Center: Evaluation of a Hospital Based Program for Continued Education in Medical Ethics. *Pediatrics*. 60:202-208, August 1977.

Lisson, Edwin. Active Medical Morals Committee: Valuable Resource for Health Care. *Hospital Progress*. 63:36, October 1982.

Lo, B., et al. Frequency of Ethical Dilemmas in Medical In-Patient Service. *Archives of Internal Medicine*. 141(8):1062-1064, July 1981.

Lobo, G. Medical Ethics Forum. *Medical Service*. 36(6): 37, 39, November-December, 1977.

MacIntyre, A. Theology, Ethics, and the Ethics of Medicine and Health Care: Comments on Papers by Novak, Mouw, Roach, Cahill, and Hart. *Journal of Medicine and Philosophy*. (4)435-443, December 4, 1979.

McCormick, R. Ethics Committees: Promise or Peril? *Law, Medicine, and Health Care*. 150-155, September 1984.

Massachusetts Law—The Substituted Judgment Doctrine Expands Beyond Life-Prolonging Decisions—In re Guardianship of Roe, 421 N.E. 2d 40 (Mass.), *Western New England Law Review*. 5:565-587, Winter 1983.

May, William. Composition and Function of Ethics Committees. *Journal of Medical Ethics*. 1:23, 1975.

Mazonson, P.D., et al. Medical Ethical Rounds: Development and Organization. *Rocky Mountain Medical Journal*. 76(6)282-288, November/December 1979.

Medical Ethics Forum—22 Models for Christian Hospitals. *Medical Service*. 38(6):23, November-December 1981.

Medical-Legal Agreement on Brain Death: An Assessment of the Uniform Determination of Death Act. *Journal of Contemporary Law*. 8:97-122, 1982.

Medical Societies Proposed Life Preservation Committees: Maryland. (N) *Hospital*. 49:227, August 1975.

Memel, S.L. The Legal Status of "No Code Orders." *Hospital Medical Staff*. 7(5):1-8, May 1978.

Middleton, Carl. A Model for Forming a Medical-Moral Committee. *Ethic Notes*. December 1981. Farmington Hills, MI: Sisters of Mercy Health Corp.

Miles, S.H., et al. The Do-Not-Resuscitate Order in a Teaching Hospital: Considerations and a Suggested Policy. *Annals of Internal Medicine*. 96(5):660-664, May 1982.

Monagle, J.F. Blueprints for Hospital Ethics Committees, *CHA Insight.* 8(20):1, June 26, 1984.

Murphy, M.A. and Murphy, J. Making Ethical Decisions Systematically. *Nursing '76.* 6:13, May 1976.

Noble, C.N. Ethics and Experts. *Hastings Center Report.* 12(3):7-15, June 1982.

Optimum Care for Hopelessly Ill Patients: A Report of the Clinical Care Committee of the Massachusetts General Hospital. *New England Journal of Medicine.* 295:362, 1976.

O'Rourke, Kevin, Ethical Committees in Hospitals. *Ethical Issues in Health Care.* IV/9, St. Louis University Medical Center, August 1983.

Paris, J.J. Terminating Treatment for Newborns: A Theological Perspective. *Law, Medicine, and Health Care.* 10(3):120,122, June 1982.

Paris, J.J., and Fletcher, A.B. Infant Doe Regulations and the Absolute Requirement to Use Nourishment and Fluids for the Dying Infant. *Law, Medicine, and Health Care.* 11(5):210, October 1983.

Pattullo, E.L. Institutional Review Boards and the Freedom to Take Risks. *New England Journal of Medicine.* 307(18):1156-1159, October 28, 1982.

Pinkus, R.L. Medical Foundations of Various Approaches to Medical-Ethic Decision-Making. *Journal of Medical Philosophy.* 6(3):295-307, August 1981.

Pope John Center Staff. "How Can Medical-Morals Committees Function Effectively in Catholic Health Facilities?" *Hospital Progress.* 64(4):77, April 1983.

President's Commission for the Study of Ethical Problems in Medicine and Biomedical and Behavioral Research. Deciding to Forego Life-Sustaining Treatment, Washington, DC: U.S. Government Printing Office, March 1983. CF index, p. 549, Ethics Committees. *Making Health Care Decisions.* p. 187.

Procaccino, J.A. Life v. Quality of Life: The Dilemma of Emerging Medical-Legal Standards. *Medical Trial Technique Quarterly.* 29(1):45-60, Summer 1982.

Rabkin, Mitchell, et al. Orders Not to Resuscitate. *New England Journal of Medicine.* 295:364, 1976.

Read, W.A. Hospital Management of Resuscitation Decisions (draft document, available from Office of Aging and Long Term Care; Hospital Research and Educational Trust, Chicago), March 1983.

Report of the ad hoc Committee on Policy for Do Not Resuscitate Decisions, Department of Medicine, Yale-New Haven Hospital, published as Levine, R.J. Do Not Resuscitate Decisions and their Implementation. *In Dilemmas of Dying.* Boston: G.K. Hall, 1981.

Report of the Surgeon General's Workshop on Children with Handicaps and Their Families. Department of Health and Human Services, DHHS Publication No. PHS—50194, December 1982.

Rescher, N. *The Allocation of Exotic Medical Lifesaving Therapy in Contemporary Issues in Bioethics.* Encino, CA: Dickenson Publishing Co., 1978.

Right to Privacy, Removal of Life-Support Systems: Leach v. Akron General Medical Center, 426 N.E. 2d 809 (Ohio), Akron Law Review 16:162-170, Summer 1982.

Robertson, J. Legal Criteria for Orders Not to Resuscitate: A Response to Justice Liacos. *Medicolegal News* 8(1):4, February 1980.

Roth, A.B., and Wild, R.A. When the Patient Refuses Treatment: Some Observations and Proposals for Handling the Difficult Case. *Saint Louis University Law Journal* 23(3):429-445, 1979.

Rothenberg, L.S., Evidentiary Hearing Required for Termination of Treatment. *Hospital Law* 13(11):3, November 1980.

Rothenberg, L.S. Are Doctors Abdicating Responsibility for Medical Treatment Decisions? *LACMA Physician* 110(16):30-32, October 1980.

Rothenberg, L.S. The Empty Search for an Imprimatur, or Delphic Oracles are in Short Supply. *Law, Medicine, and Health Care* 10(3):115-116, June 1982.

Sargeant, K.J. Withholding Treatment from Defective Newborns: Substituted Judgment, Informed Consent, and the Quinlan Decision. *Gonzaga Law Review* 13:781-811, 1978.

Scott, R.S. Life Support: Who Decides? How? *Legal Aspects of Medical Practice* 7(10):33-36, October 1979.

Shannon, T.A. What Guidance From the Guidelines? *Hastings Center Report* 7:28, March 1977.

Shannon, T.A. The Withdrawal of Treatment: The Costs of Benefits of Guidelines. In *Bioethics: Basic Writings on the Key Ethical Questions that Surround the Major Modern Biological Possibilities and Problems.* T.A. Shannon, Ed. Ramsey, NJ: Paulist Press, revised 1981.

Showalter, J.S. Determining Death: The Legal and Theological Aspects of Brain-Related Criteria. *Catholic Lawyer.* 27:112-28, Spring 1982.

Siegler, M. Decision-Making Strategy for Clinical-ethical Problems in Medicine. *Archives of Internal Medicine.* 142(12):2178-2179, November 1982.

Somfai, Bela. Moral Leadership in a Socialized Health Care System. (Part II) *CHAC Review.* 8(1):24-6, January-February 1980.

Stalder, G. Ethical Committees in a Pediatric Hospital. *European Journal of Pediatrics.* 136(2): 22, May 1981.

Stevens, J.E. Hospital Ethics Committees. *Quality Review Bulletin.* 9(6):162-63, June 1983.

Strong, C. The Tiniest Newborns. *Hastings Center Report.* 13(4):14-19, Fall 1983.

Sullivan, L.J. The How and Why of Ethics Committees. *CHAC Review.* 12(3):8-10, Autumn 1984.

Teel, Karen. The Physician's Dilemma, A Doctor's View: What the Law Should Be. *Baylor Law Review.* 27:609, Winter 1975.

Van Leeuwen, G. Natural Committee for Life: Accepting Death in Our Patients. *Clinical Pediatrics.* 12(2):64-65, December 1973.

Veatch, Robert. Courts, Committees, and Caring. *American Medical News.* 23(20) pp. 1, 2, 11-13, May 23, 1980.

Veatch, Robert. Hospital Ethics Committees: Is There a Role? *Hastings Center Report*. 7:22, March 1977.

Veatch, Robert. What is the Scope of Hospital Ethics Committees? *Hospital Medical Staff*. 6:24, Summer 1977.

Wallice-Barnhill, G.R., et al. Medical, Legal and Ethical Issues in Critical Care. *Critical Care Medicine*. 10:57, 1982.

Weisman, S.A. Nursing Home Experience with an Ethics Committee. *Nursing Homes*. 29(5):2-4, September-October 1980.

Westervelt, F.B. The Selection Process as Viewed from Within: A Reply to Childress. In *Ethics and Health Care Policy*. R.M. Veatch, R. Brawson, Eds., Cambridge, MA: Ballinger Publishing Co., 1976.

Wussburg, C., and Hartz, J.N. Legal, Ethical Risks Made Doctors Hesitant to Stop Life Support Systems. *Healthcare Review*. 12(6):64,66,68-69, December 1979/January 1980.

Youngner, Stuart, et al. A National Survey of Hospital Ethics Committees. In President's Commission for the Study of Ethical Problems in Medicine and Biomedical and Behavioral Research. Deciding to Forego Life-Sustaining Treatment, Washington, DC: U.S. Government Printing Office, March 1983.

Youngner, Stuart. Patients' Attitudes Toward Hospital Ethics Committees. *Law, Medicine, and Health Care*. 12(1):21-25, February 1984.

State of New Jersey Guidelines for Health Care Facilities to Implement Procedures Concerning the Care of Comatose Non-Cognitive Patients (undated) [10-1005].

Statement of the Bio-Medical Ethics Committee: Hennepin County Medical Center on the Case of Sergeant David Mack (June 23, 1980) [7-169].

Appendix II
Resources: Books and Journals

Beauchamp, T., and Childress, J. *Principles of Biomedical Ethics*. New York: Oxford University Press, 1979.

> A clear concise textbook explaining basic ethical principles and showing how they are applied to major issues in bioethics such as informed consent, risk/benefit assessment, confidentiality, and decisions to terminate therapy. Cases and codes of ethics are included.

Beauchamp, T., and Walters, L. *Contemporary Issues in Bioethics*. 2d ed. Belmont, CA: Wadsworth Publishing Co., 1982.

> An anthology of important essays dealing with such topics as ethical theory, concepts of health and disease, patients' rights and professional responsibilities, abortion, euthanasia, allocation of medical resources, and research.

Benton, G. *Death and Dying: Principles and Practices in Patient Care*. New York: Van Nostrand Reinhold, 1978.

Bioethics: Basic Writings on the Key Ethical Questions that Surround the Major, Modern Biological Possibilities and Problems. T.A. Shannon, Ed. Ramsey, NJ: Paulist Press, 1981.

Biomedical Ethics and the Law. J.M. Humber, R.F. Almeder, eds. New York: Plenum Press, 1979.

Biomedical Ethics Reviews, 1983. J.M. Humber, R.F. Almeder, eds., Clifton, NJ: Humana Press, 1983.

Brody, H. *Ethical Decisions in Medicine*. Boston: Little-Brown Co., 1981.

Childress, J. *Who Should Decide? Paternalism in Health Care*. New York: Oxford University Press, 1982.

Contemporary Issues in Bioethics. T.L. Beauchamp, L.R. Walters, eds. Encino, CA: Dickenson Publishing Co., 1978.

Death Inside Out: The Hastings Center Report. P. Steinfels, R.M. Veatch, eds. New York: Harper & Row Publishers, 1975.

Encyclopedia of Bioethics. W. Reich, ed. New York: The Free Press, 1978.

Ethical Issues in Death and Dying. R.F. Weir, ed. New York: Columbia University Press, 1977.

Ethical Issues Relating to Life and Death. J. Ladd, ed. New York: Oxford University Press, 1977.

The Ethics of Resource Allocation in Health Care. K.M. Boyd, ed. Edinburgh, Scotland: Edinburgh University Press, 1979.

Fox R. and Swazey, J., *The Courage to Fail: A Social View of Organ Transplants and Dialysis*. Chicago: University of Chicago, 1974.

Frontiers in Medical Ethics: Applications in a Medical Setting. V. Abernathy, ed. Cambridge, MA: Ballinger Publishing Co., 1980.

Harron, F., Burnside, J., and Beauchamp, T. *Health and Human Values: A Guide to Making Your Own Decisions*. New Haven, CT: Yale University Press, 1982.

> The authors explore such issues as euthanasia, abortion, in vitro fertilization, health care and distributive justice, truth telling and informed consent, determination of death, and genetic engineering. There are two very practical companion volumes: *Human Values in Medicine and Health Care: Audio/Visual Resources*. Approximately 400 audiovisual items are listed. Most are annotated and all provide information about purchase and rental. *Biomedical and Ethical Issues: A Digest of Law and Policy Development*. This handbook contains excerpts and summaries of influential court decisions, state and federal legislation, and federal guidelines, as well as policy statements from various religious and professional organizations regarding developments in the practice of health care.

Jacobovits, I. *Jewish Medical Ethics*. New York: Block Publishing Co., 1975.

Jonsen, A., Seigler, M., and Winslade, W. *Clinical Ethics: A Practical Approach to Ethical Decisions in Clinical Medicine*. New York: MacMillan Publishing Co., 1982.

> This is an excellent and unusual book, which approaches clinical decision making from a case-based approach. It will be especially helpful for the clinician. The authors include a comprehensive bibliography at the end of each chapter.

Katz, J. and Capron, A.M. *Catastrophic Diseases: Who Decides What?* New York: Russell Sage Foundation, 1975.

Kieffer, G.H. *Bioethics: A Textbook of Issues*. Reading, MA: Addison-Wesley Publishing Company, 1979.

Killing and Letting Die. B. Steinbock, ed., Englewood Cliffs, NJ, Prentice Hall, 1980.

Legal and Ethical Aspects of Treating Critically and Terminally Ill Patients. A.E. Doudera, and J.D. Peters, eds. Ann Arbor, MI: AUPHA Press, 1982.

McCormick, R. *How Brave a New World?* New York: Doubleday, 1981.

Medical Ethics: A Clinical Textbook and Reference for the Health Professions. N. Abrams, and M.D. Buckner, eds. Cambridge, MA: Unit Press, 1983.

Medical Treatment of the Dying: Moral Issues. M.D. Bayles, D.M. High, eds. Cambridge, MA: Schenkman Publishing Co., Inc., 1978.

Meyers, D.W. *Medico-Legal Implications of Death and Dying*. New York: Lawyers Co-operative Publishing Co., 1981.

Morasczewski, A.S. and Showalter, J.S. *Determination of Death: Theological, Medical, Ethical, and Legal Issues*. St. Louis, The Catholic Health Association of the United States, 1982.

Presidents Commission for the Study of Ethical Problems in Medicine and Behavioral Research, *Deciding to Forego Life Sustaining Treatment (1983)*; *Making Healthcare Decisions 1982*; *Defining Death 1981.* Washington, DC: U.S. Government Printing Office.

Robertson, J.A. *The Rights of the Critically Ill.* Cambridge, MA: Ballinger Publishing Co., 1983.

Shapiro, M.H., and Spece, R.G., Jr. *Cases, Materials, and Problems on Bioethics·and Law.* Saint Paul, MN: West Publishing Co., 1981.

Veatch, R. *Case Studies in Medical Ethics.* Boston: Harvard University Press, 1977.

> For those who do not have enough cases to discuss, this will supply them. Topics include health care delivery, duties to patients, confidentiality, truth telling, abortion, genetics, experimentation, and death and dying.

Veatch, R. *Death, Dying and the Biological Revolution.* New Haven, CT: Yale University Press, 1976.

> This book treats the ethical issues surrounding the care of the dying in a comprehensive way. It is, for the most part, a good summary statement of current thinking on these issues.

Veatch, R. *A Theory of Medical Ethics.* New York: Basic Books, Inc., 1981.

> The author notes that traditional codes of medical ethics are not adequate to the ethical problems in medicine today. He attempts to develop a more comprehensive theory of medical ethics and apply it to clinical cases.

Walton, D.N. *Ethics of Withdrawal of Life-Support Systems: Case Studies on Decision Making in Intensive Care.* Westport, CT: Greenwood Press, 1983.

Wong, C., and Swazey, J. *Dilemmas of Dying: Policies and Procedures for Decisions Not to Treat.* Boston: G.K. Hall, Medical Publishers, 1981.

> This book, the result of a conference, explores the medical, moral, legal, and procedural aspects of nontreatment decisions. It is practical and in many cases creative.

Journals

Hastings Center Report. (Published bimonthly.) Institute of Society, Ethics and the Life Sciences, 360 Broadway, Hastings-on-Hudson, NY 10706.

American Journal of Law and Medicine. (Quarterly.) American Society of Law and Medicine, 765 Commonwealth Ave., Boston, MA 02215.

Law, Medicine & Health Care. (Published six times a year.) American Society of Law and Medicine, 765 Commonwealth Ave., Boston, MA 02215.

Lineacre Quarterly, A Journal of the Philosophy and Ethics of Medical Practice. (Quarterly.) The National Federation of Catholic Physicians Guilds, 850 Elm Grove Rd., Elm Grove, WI 53122.

Journal of Medicine and Philosophy. *Society for Health and Human Values.* (Quarterly.) University of Chicago Press, 5801 Ellis Ave., Chicago, IL 60637.

The following medical journals frequently have articles on ethical issues in medicine:

New England Journal of Medicine Annals of Internal Medicine
Journal of the American Medical Association

■ Appendix III
Resources:
Bibliographical Listings

BioethicsLine. National Library of Medical Data Base, Medlars Management. *BioethicsLine* provides bibliographic information on questions of ethics and public policy arising in health care or biomedical research. Developed at the Center for Bioethics, Kennedy Institute of Ethics, Georgetown University. *BioethicsLine* contains English language citations to material published from 1973 to the present. It is available through most libraries.

Bibliography of Bioethics. Yearly volumes that contain material available through BioethicsLine. Gayle Research Co., Detroit, MI 48226.

Bibliography of Society, Ethics and the Life Sciences. Institute of Society, Ethics and the Life Sciences. Hastings-on-Hudson, NY 10706. Issued annually.

New Titles in Bioethics. Published monthly by the Center for Bioethics, Kennedy Institute of Ethics, Georgetown University, Washington, DC 20057. A listing of recent acquisitions by the Bioethics Library at the Kennedy Institute.